Control and Eradication of Endemic Infectious Diseases in Cattle

Control and Eradication of Endemic Infectious Diseases in Cattle

Hans Houe

Liza Rosenbaum Nielsen

Søren Saxmose Nielsen

Disclaimer:

The approach and advice offered in this book are intended to be general in nature and should not be used to substitute herd-specific advisory services. The presentation of the framework and the individual elements of disease control covered in this book are intended to encourage and support the development of successful disease control programmes, but should always be used with careful consideration for local or regional societal circumstances.

Please note that some resources, such as websites, are referred to in this book for the convenience of readers, and are not managed by the authors. We do not review, control or take responsibility for the content of these resources.

© Individual author and College Publications 2014. All rights reserved. The authors have contributed equally to the book

ISBN 978-1-84890-156-8

College Publications
Scientific Director: Dov Gabbay
Managing Director: Jane Spurr

http://www.collegepublications.co.uk

Cover designed by Laraine Welch
Printed by Lightning Source, Milton Keynes, UK

Table of Contents

List of abbreviations

AP	Apparent prevalence
BTM	Bulk tank milk
BVDV	Bovine virus diarrhoea virus
CFU	Colony forming units
CP	Cytopathic
IgG	Immunoglobulin G
IFN-γ	Interferon-γ
MAP	*Mycobacterium avium* subsp. *paratuberculosis*
NCP	Non-cytopathic
ODC	Optical density corrected (corrected for negative controls)
PI	Persistently infected (a term used specifically for BVDV-PI animals)
S. Dublin	*Salmonella enterica* subsp. *enterica* serovar Dublin
Se	(Diagnostic) Sensitivity
Sp	(Diagnostic) Specificity
TP	True prevalence
YS	Young stock

Preface

For the past 15-20 years, the authors of this book have been involved in the research and development of control and eradication programmes for three different diseases within the Danish cattle industry. The programmes for the individual diseases evolved at their own pace according to the specific traits of the pathogens concerned, and the socioeconomic circumstances. Throughout the years, different stakeholders have often anticipated that experiences from control efforts of one disease could be transferred to another. This was sometimes possible, but often to a surprisingly limited extent. We believe that this inability to generalise between the programmes is to some extent due to the lack of a common template for describing the preconditions for disease eradication, and an exhaustive list of the important elements that make up successful disease control and eradication programmes.

The aim of this book is to describe the key elements in systematic disease control and eradication efforts for future development of new programmes. Furthermore, it is useful to consider this template of key elements when reading existing literature, in order to reveal apparent knowledge gaps to be addressed or investigated further. This book aims to reach a broad group of readers, including: students; professionals in veterinary practice, industry and governmental institutions; researchers; and others involved in control and eradication of endemic diseases in livestock.

We would like to acknowledge the discussions with our many colleagues from different institutions and organisations over the past many years. We also express our gratitude to Sarah Layhe for an excellent job in proofreading of this book.

Frederiksberg, 2014

Hans Houe, Liza Rosenbaum Nielsen and Søren Saxmose Nielsen

1

Introduction

There are several historical examples of successful control and regional eradication of infectious diseases in cattle. Diseases affecting cattle health which have been eradicated from Denmark include: bovine tuberculosis, enzootic bovine leukosis, infectious bovine rhinotracheitis, bovine virus diarrhoea, brucellosis and foot-and-mouth disease. From the first speculation of it being a feasible option, the period of time taken to achieve eradication was dependent on the disease in question, and varied between a few years up to several decades. Before the decision to eradicate was made, there were usually strong arguments both for and against eradication. It was not always clear when sufficient evidence existed to deem eradication feasible and advantageous. Therefore, there is a need to provide a more systematic framework to support decision-making before, during, and after the establishment of eradication programmes.

There are many explanations as to why the progression of eradication is different from one disease to another. The available knowledge about the nature of the infectious agent, its transmission routes, and the available tools for eradication vary considerably over time. Moreover, the variation in occurrence, pathogenesis and spread mechanisms vary between individual diseases, requiring different approaches to be used for different diseases. Eradication of diseases also progresses differently between countries as a reflection of the variation in socioeconomic conditions, size and structure of animal populations, reservoirs and the nature of the farming industries, as well as national and international markets. However, despite the differences between various diseases and their management in the countries in which they occur, it is possible to establish some common principles for effective approaches based on past experiences. These principles consist of a variety of elements including: motivation among stakeholders; availability of efficient biosecurity measures and test-strategies; feasibility in practice; adequate resources and infrastructure; as well as sufficient education of the parties involved. It is crucial to consider how these elements evolve over time, and when there is sufficient support to determine that eradication can be achieved. During the eradication programme, additional important information and critical issues often arise, which must also be addressed for the programme to be successful in all stages.

The objective of this book is therefore twofold. Firstly, it will describe the content of the individual elements of a control and eradication programme. Secondly, it will discuss how the individual elements can be compiled to constitute sufficient grounds for deciding, planning and carrying out eradication programmes for endemic infectious diseases in cattle.

Usually, eradication programmes are preceded by a control programme aiming to reduce the prevalence of the disease. Therefore, the term 'control programme' is also used throughout the book, but most often with the inherent long-term scope of eradication. The definitions of control and eradication are described in more detail in Chapter 2. As the endemic infection will eventually become an exotic infection after it has been eradicated from the given population, preparedness for that situation will also briefly be touched upon. However, the main focus of this book is the eradication process of endemic diseases.

Some chapters of the textbook focus on individual elements, whereas others compile information from several elements, in particular the chapters on ultimately taking the decision to initiate an eradication programme (Chapter 8) and on follow-up investigations during the eradication phase (Chapter 10). We attempt to follow the thought processes of decision makers, who will usually start by evaluating the importance of the infection, and thereafter explore the more technical matters. If eradication is deemed possible and justifiable, the feasibility in practice is considered, together with the capacity in the society, including resources and educational competences.

Throughout the textbook, selected diseases will be used as examples. In particular, the three infectious agents: bovine virus diarrhoea virus (BVDV); *Salmonella* Dublin (*S.* Dublin); and *Mycobacterium avium* subsp.

paratuberculosis (MAP) will be used as recurring examples in the chapters, as they have been subjects of intensive research by each of the authors (BVDV by H Houe, *S.* Dublin by LR Nielsen and MAP by SS Nielsen), and because we have been involved in the implementation and establishment of control and eradication programmes for these infections. Specific details on these infections are compiled in Chapter 11, which can be read separately or used as reference when reading the other chapters. By using examples of diseases, the book establishes a common framework for disease eradication. However, we have restricted the amount of arguments in order to keep the general overview of the topic. The basic idea behind the book is that for each disease, it is possible to establish a certain profile governed by the agent characteristics and its interaction with the host and environment. The profile determines which control elements must be taken into consideration. It is important to stress that every eradication programme is a learning process in itself, and individual consideration must be given both to the characteristics of the disease and to the specific societal and livestock sector contexts in each country.

By applying the analytical approach and trying to establish a general overview, it is our hope that this book reaches a broad group of readers, including: students; professionals in veterinary practice, industry and governmental institutions; researchers; and others involved in the control and eradication of endemic diseases in livestock.

2

The need for a systematic approach for disease control and eradication of endemic diseases

2.1. Introduction

Animal populations that have not been exposed to specific pathogens and that have not been vaccinated, are often much more susceptible to infection than animals that have been exposed to the endemic pathogens. A failing eradication programme can therefore have devastating effects on the many herds that have become partly or fully susceptible during the initial phases of the programme. Therefore, a systematic approach for successful disease control and eradication is required.

It is sometimes argued that it is preferable to preserve immunity in the population by living with a pathogen, rather than having a naïve and vulnerable population. On the other hand, if eradication is possible, it may very well be a waste of money to have continual expenditures and losses due to the infection, without any progress towards eradication. Furthermore, animal health and welfare (and sometimes food safety) may be generally better, and new trade markets may open if specific pathogens are absent. Therefore, a decision to aim for eradication is often relevant, but must rely on some evidence that it is possible. This chapter provides a list of the prerequisites and elements required for effective disease control aiming at eradication. Moreover, it provides definitions and terminology used in such programmes.

2.2. Research history on BVDV

To illustrate the complexity of information, a simplified diagram of the research history of BVDV infection from the first detection of disease in 1946 (Olafson et al., 1946) until its eradication in some countries approximately 60 years later (Moennig et al., 2005; Sandvik, 2004) is illustrated in Fig. 2.1.

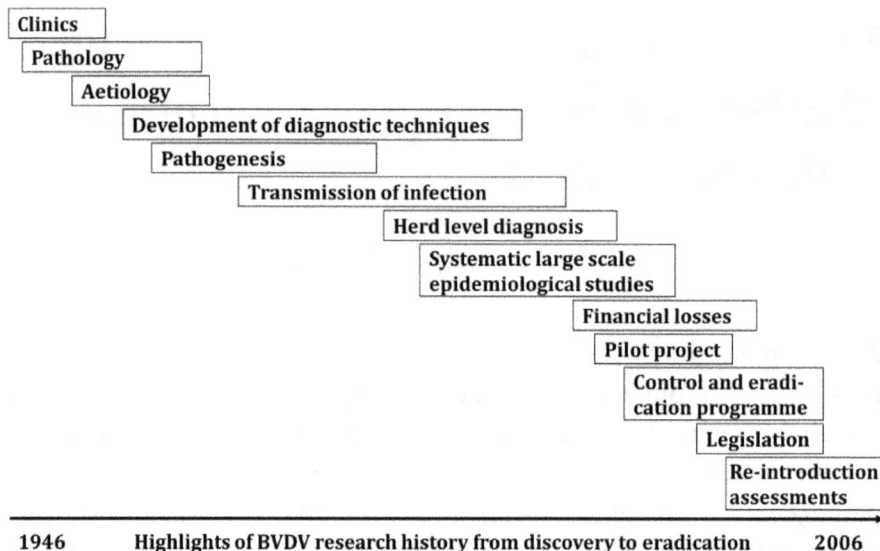

| Clinics |
| Pathology |
| Aetiology |
| Development of diagnostic techniques |
| Pathogenesis |
| Transmission of infection |
| Herd level diagnosis |
| Systematic large scale epidemiological studies |
| Financial losses |
| Pilot project |
| Control and eradication programme |
| Legislation |
| Re-introduction assessments |

| 1946 | Highlights of BVDV research history from discovery to eradication | 2006 |

Figure 2.1. Schematic and simplified diagram of the main topics in the research history of BVDV infection.

It is useful to consider the case of BVDV as an example of the general trends in progression through the steps of disease research. The first reports often consist of short case stories describing clinical and pathological findings. Hereafter, identification and characterisation of the aetiological agent is performed, followed by development of diagnostic techniques to detect the agent and the ensuing immune responses. The clinical, pathological and laboratory findings are interpreted together, in order to elucidate the pathogenesis of infection, such as transient and persistent infection with BVDV. Experimental studies and infection models are used to document the aetiology, demonstrate important transmission routes between animals, and to further elaborate on the understanding of the pathogenesis. Typically at a later stage, when good laboratory techniques are established, large-scale epidemiological studies are undertaken to investigate the occurrence of infection and identify risk factors for transmission of infection, as well as risk factors that may aggravate the infection. Models of the spread of infectious agents in relevant populations help us to understand and identify critical control points in control programmes,

6

and intervention studies or small-scale control trials are often carried out to test the effect and feasibility at some of these critical control points in practice. Large epidemiological studies create the foundation for estimating the importance of infection, which is often expressed in financial terms, but which may also be expressed as the importance for animal welfare or public health. Each of these research findings are important elements in the decision-making process for eradication, but may also contribute to the eradication programme itself.

Despite some sequential trends in these research approaches, they may in practice be done more or less in parallel. However, from an eradication point of view, they can be seen as a 'chain' of elements that all need to be sufficiently addressed to plan a systematic and effective programme. In addition to all the information obtained from disciplines of natural science and economics applied to animal health shown in Fig 2.1, a number of aspects from social sciences are required. Communication with farmers and farmers' organisations is of great importance in order to understand perceptions and potential compliance issues, as well as to obtain sufficient and necessary incentives. In addition, organisational structure is crucial so that testing can be performed at reliable laboratories, herd classification can occur using a common and accepted grouping system, and general advice for farmers can be given efficiently by trained advisors. In the later stages of a programme, the inclusion of legislation is necessary as there will invariably be some farmers who do not want to participate in voluntary programmes, and their herds will become a risk to those free from the infection. For example, before the BVDV eradication programme in Denmark was initiated, some farmers deliberately kept PI animals in their herds to maintain high immunity, whereas other farmers tried to get rid of the PI animals. Such a non-systematic approach will mean that neighbouring farms can have a very different infection status and that the infection status of nearby herds is unknown. An important reason why there is a need for a systematic approach is that just one weak link in the whole chain of elements can hamper the entire programme.

2.3. Definition of control and eradication
Quite a number of definitions of control and eradication of diseases have been given in the literature. In this context, dealing with endemic infectious diseases, we find the definitions given by Andrews and

Langmuir (1963) most useful. They define control as 'the purposeful reduction of specific disease prevalence to relatively low level of occurrence, though transmission occurs frequently enough to prevent its permanent disappearance'. For eradication, they add to reduction of specific disease prevalence that it is 'to the point of continued absence of transmission within a specified area.' In practice, eradication means a prevalence close to zero for continued absence of transmission to be realised.

These definitions have several advantages when it comes to establishing operational programmes. The definition of control as 'relatively low level of occurrence' may seem vague, but it would not be practical to give an arbitrary prevalence of, for example, 5% as the aim for a control programme due to the substantial variation between diseases. The definition of eradication gives room for the possibility that the disease agent may actually still be present, e.g. in the environment or wildlife. However, providing the transmission of infection is brought to a complete stop, this definition is found to be sufficient. It is also more realistic to aim for eradication in a specified area (often a country) since global eradication is very rare (although it has been achieved for rinderpest). For such rare events, we can reserve the term 'global eradication'. We are aware that some suggest the word eradication to mean global eradication, but we prefer the traditional terminology, as it is the most consistent in existing literature.

To emphasise the importance of monitoring the progress of programmes, it has been suggested to distinguish between 'systematic' and 'non-systematic' control programmes (Lindberg and Houe, 2005; Moennig et al., 2005). The non-systematic approach refers to any intervention decided on an individual herd basis without monitoring or evaluation. Systematic control refers to a goal-oriented reduction in prevalence and incidence, where the progress is monitored and evaluated and the programme is controlled from a central organisational body such as the veterinary authorities or an industrial organisation. Obviously, the systematic approach with monitoring is necessary in eradication programmes.

In this textbook, the concept of disease control is used with the long-term objective of eradication. Therefore, the use of a systematic approach is most useful as surveillance helps to provide the tools for the final aim of eradication. It also helps to rationalise the use of vaccination as part of an eradication programme. Thus, if vaccines are used in conjunction with close monitoring, they can be helpful in the initial phases to reduce the prevalence of some infections. The long term objective of eradication also implies that control programmes not aiming at eradication (e.g. mastitis) are outside the scope of this book.

2.4. The prerequisites of a systematic approach for disease control and eradication

A systematic approach for disease control and eradication can be seen as a broad framework for the activities. Similar frameworks have previously been referred to as 'preconditions and criteria for deciding upon eradication' (Yekutiel, 1980) or a 'constellation of conditions that make eradication of infectious diseases feasible' (Dowdle and Cochi, 2011). They include elements from both natural and social sciences, as well as politics and even religion. For example, Box 2.1 lists the preconditions and criteria suggested by Yekutiel (1980). The framework must establish the best evidence by combining scientific knowledge with practical experience and present conditions and constraints in the relevant region.

Box 2.1. Preconditions and criteria for deciding upon eradication (Cited from Yekutiel, 1980)

---

1. There should be a main tool (control measure), completely effective in breaking transmission, simple in application and relatively inexpensive
2. The disease should have epidemiological features facilitating effective case detection and surveillance in the advanced stages of the programme
3. The disease must be of recognised socioeconomic importance, national or international
4. There should be a specific reason for eradication – rather than control – of the disease
5. Resources: finance, administration, manpower, health services
6. Socio-ecological conditions

The list of preconditions and criteria outlined in Box 2.1 will be elaborated upon further in this book.

As with most activities in the world, the very first criterion to be considered is whether there is any motivation or a driver for the activity. Therefore, although motivation is listed third in Box 2.1 we will use it as a starting point. The motivation often appears before it is based on exact quantifiable measures. Thus, for many diseases it is apparent from an early stage that they cause considerable production losses, severe pain in the animals or that they have a zoonotic potential.

If the disease does not have any severe impact on any of these 'values', it will not be prioritised. However, some diseases may have a somewhat 'hidden' impact and therefore efforts should be made to quantify these effects so that everyone has a common understanding of the motivation. Thus, the initial thoughts about disease eradication are mostly related to values. Other important criteria are more technical in character. In particular, how easy it will be to prevent the spread of infection. If sufficient biosecurity measures are difficult to establish, then their creation may be considered a constraint to the farming business (e.g. if free trade is not possible). For almost all diseases it is technically possible to establish sufficiently rigorous biosecurity measures to prevent transmission, but the price may seem too high. The biosecurity measures can certainly not stand alone, because it is an activity that will always be adjusted to the practical and economic circumstances. Biosecurity measures are also related to the technical possibilities of having an efficient test-strategy. A test-strategy may include testing of individual animals in order to issue certificates for animal trade, but in particular, also testing for herd classification and monitoring. Many of these technical criteria are concerned with building up enough scientific evidence so that transmission can be prevented and surveillance is efficient. Yet in addition to scientific evidence, proof-of-concept in practice may also be needed. This can be based on pilot studies or 'feasibility studies', where the efficiency of experimentally proven biosecurity measures can also be tested in practice. If feasibility studies also support that eradication is possible, a plan for the programme can be made. Importantly, the plan should take into account whether the society has sufficient resources such as laboratory capacity and that there is sufficient determination to comply with guidelines and legislation accompanying the programme.

The necessary requirements are organised in the following topics (covered in Chapters 3-10 in this book):

Chapter 3: Motivation – socioeconomic aspects

Chapter 4: Biosecurity: actions to mitigate transmission of infectious diseases

Chapter 5: Establishment of purpose-specific and systematic test-strategies

Chapter 6: The pilot study

Chapter 7: Resources

Chapter 8: Deciding upon the initiation of a systematic control and eradication programme

Chapter 9: Communication

Chapter 10: Follow-up investigations and adjustments of the eradication programme

The decision-making process for the initiation, planning and organisation of an eradication programme is very complex, as the necessary information must be compiled from many different sources. Over the years, there are many different steps and levels of decisions required as a programme is modified according to new knowledge obtained, and to the progress of the programme itself. Whereas the scientific knowledge on many individual biological and economic elements is usually published in detail, a description of the full process of an eradication programme is often lacking or fragmented. In Chapter 11, the knowledge and experiences from control and eradication programmes for three different diseases have been compiled systematically under the headlines of the necessary elements of such programmes.

References

Andrews JM and Langmuir AD: 1963, The philosophy of disease eradication. American Journal of Public Health 53: 1-6.

Dowdle WR, Cochi SL, 2011. The principles and feasibility of disease eradication. Vaccine 29 (Supp. 4): D70-D73.

Moennig V, Houe H, Lindberg A, 2005. BVD control in Europe: Current status and perspectives. Animal Health Research Reviews 6: 63-74.

Lindberg A, Houe H, 2005 Characteristics in BVDV epidemiology of relevance to control. Preventive Veterinary Medicine 72: 55-73.

Olafson P, MacCallum AD, Fox FH, 1946. An apparently new transmissible disease of cattle. Cornell Veterinarian 36: 205-213.

Sandvik T, 2004. Progress of control and prevention programs for bovine viral diarrhea virus in Europe. Veterinary Clinics of North America. Food Animal Practice 20: 151-169.

Yekutiel P, 1980, Eradication of infectious diseases: a critical study. *In*: Contribution to epidemiology and biostatistics, vol. 2, Karger, Basel, Switzerland.

3

Motivation - Socioeconomic aspects

3.1. Introduction

Incentives to comply with plans and guidelines are crucial at all stakeholder levels - from farmers to government - in any control or eradication programme. Sufficient biological knowledge concerning biosecurity and test-strategies for a successful eradication programme may be present, but if evident and visible incentives are not in place, the programme is unlikely to succeed. A benefit based on financial gain has often been used as the main argument for a more systematic investment in disease programmes. Likewise, increased food safety has been a primary benefit, and in recent years, an increased focus on animal welfare has made the evaluation and implementation of incentives much more complex. Different stakeholders would prioritise profit maximisation, animal welfare and food safety to different degrees. These priorities are often deeply rooted in society as they may be related to specific traditions or general ethical debates. Therefore, a control or eradication programme that has been successful in one country may not be transferrable to another country without considering the socioeconomic aspects.

This chapter will outline the principles for establishing incentives, including calculation of economic costs, different types of cost-benefit analyses and assessment of animal welfare and food safety. Concerning details on topics such as approaches to and methodologies of economic analyses and welfare assessments, the reader is referred to other textbooks, as it is not the intention to cover these areas as such, but to include them only in the context of disease control and eradication. Thresholds at which incentives are considered sufficient are discussed, together with examples from different disease control programmes. The chapter essentially aims to address the question: 'Why should we initiate a systematic control or eradication programme?'

3.2. Economic costs

Economics has been defined as, 'the study of making rational choices/decisions in the allocation of scarce resources for the achievement of competing goals' (Rushton, 2009). Thus, it is a basis for making decisions e.g. by calculating how the best return is obtained from a given investment. Returns and investments can include very different measures such as money, leisure time, animal welfare, prestige and product quality. However, for simplicity, a starting point here will include measures that can directly or indirectly be expressed in monetary terms.

Calculations of return of investment or cost-benefit analyses can be relatively complex. Therefore, it can be a good starting point simply to calculate the economic costs resulting from the infection at a given stage at herd and sector level. The economic costs give an indication of the theoretical maximum amount of money that can possibly be gained. Although it may not be possible to obtain the full amount (e.g. due to measures that cannot be expressed in monetary terms), calculation of economic costs has often been an important motivation to initiate new control measures.

The economic costs from diseases in the cattle production systems consist of direct losses in production such as milk, meat and live-born calves as well as expenditure due to treatment and prophylaxis. Note that even if there is not a formal control programme in place, some activities and hence expenditure for the handling of diseased animals will still be necessary. In this context, we use the terminology that economic costs consist of the sum of the production losses and expenditures (Bennett et al., 1999; McInerney et al., 1992):

Economic cost = Production losses + Expenditures

For many of the important diseases, there are lots of studies and reports on the associated economic costs. The different study types include:

a) Case reports on disease outbreaks;
b) Systematic calculations based on observational epidemiological studies in larger populations where the calculations can be made as, for example, average costs per cow;
c) Simulation studies aggregating information input from other types of studies.

Although the most relevant figure is the economic cost, quite often only the economic losses are provided. Therefore in the following, the term 'losses' is often used, in particular if it is unclear whether both losses and expenditures; or only losses were included in the calculations.

Case reports on losses from disease outbreaks
One might think that it would be the average losses that were most relevant for the decision to initiate a control programme, but case reports of outbreaks in individual herds can have a high impact from a motivational point of view. A primary reason is that case reports represent an actual scenario to which a decision maker can directly relate. The case may represent an extreme situation, but the farmer and his advisors can provide first-hand experiences from the outbreak to others, and for some people will therefore have high credibility. Thus, some diseases may on average only have moderate economic impact, but knowing that the infection can occasionally have a devastating effect on the individual farm makes case reports highly relevant, even though they may only be representative of the worst cases of outbreaks.

For BVDV infections, an outline of various studies showed that the economic losses due to 'initial outbreaks' could vary from approximately EUR 20 to 600 per cow present in a herd (Saatkamp et al., 2006). An 'initial outbreak' means an outbreak occurring in a BVDV naïve herd. Variation in the reported costs can be due to biological variation in the virulence of the pathogen or management of the population (and hence the severity of the outbreak) but it can also be caused by differences in how many elements are included in the economic calculations in different studies. Hence, sometimes only the most direct losses from diseased and dead animals are included,

15

whereas in other studies production losses from reduced milk production, as well as treatment costs are also included. Case reports are usually not representative of the population, so it does not make sense to calculate average economic costs from these figures. However, the calculated figures show that under some circumstances the infection can have devastating effects in individual herds.

Observational and theoretical studies estimating the average losses at herd level or higher

Losses calculated in the so-called outbreak situation will only be representative (or 'true') for a relatively short time period. Hereafter, the herd may gradually become immune and the losses reduced (Nielsen et al., 2013). For many infections, a herd will continue to be endemically infected; either by continuous presence of the infection in the herd, or by relatively frequent reintroduction after the herd has been cleared. In order to estimate the true long-term economic effect of diseases in endemic areas, many studies have included empirical data on production losses and other costs of disease, into different types of models. For BVDV infections, the average loss per cow in more or less endemically infected herds has been estimated in the range between EUR 30 and 60 (Saatkamp et al., 2006). At the national level, the figures will be somewhat lower as some herds will stay free of infection for longer periods. For BVDV infections, summaries of studies have concluded losses in the range of USD 10-40 per calving (Houe, 2003) or as narrow as EUR 15-20 (Saatkamp et al., 2006). Note that at national level, the annual losses are often given per calving in the herds. This is approximately the same as losses per cow anticipating that a cow has one calf per year.

3.3. Using cost estimations as motivation for eradication
Both the losses calculated in the outbreak situation as well as the average losses per animal have been used as 'drivers' to motivate support of eradication programmes. For example, knowing that BVDV infections may cause an abortion storm and very high mortality can be extremely motivating for risk-averse farmers. Communication of such information may encourage more farmers to comply with the guidelines of the programme.

16

At sector level, the average losses can be highly motivating for the cattle industry by showing the potential gain, and hence indicate the extent of financial resources that can be invested in a control programme.

3.4. Optimisation of decisions – Cost-benefit analysis

The basic principle for optimising decisions on an economic basis is the loss-expenditure frontier (Fig. 3.1). In short, the principle is that investments in disease control should continue as long as EUR 1 of investment (control expenditure) gives more than EUR 1 in return due to reduced production losses (solid curve in Fig. 3.1). Put differently: the total economic impact, including both production losses and control expenditures (the sum of the vertical and horizontal dashed line in Fig. 3.1), should be minimised (McInerney et al., 1992). This is illustrated where the oblique line touches the curve (at the dot in Fig. 3.1).

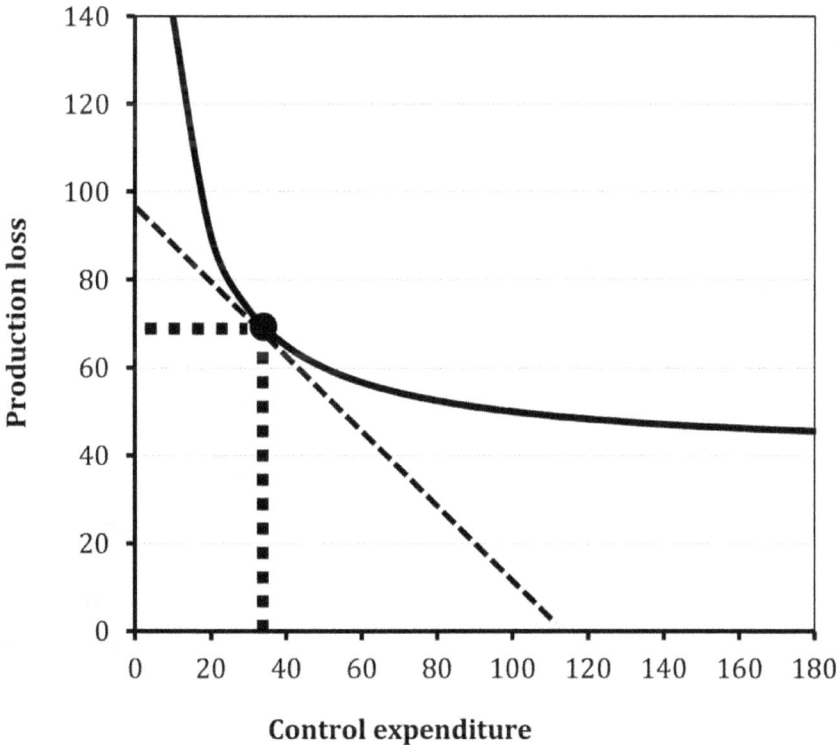

Figure 3.1. The principle of the loss-expenditure frontier for optimising expenditures for disease control.

Among the available techniques for determining the optimal decision, the cost-benefit analysis has been widely used (Rushton, 2009). Cost refers in this context to control expenditures and benefit refers to reduction in losses. The cost-benefit analysis is advantageous as it accounts for the fact that the return from an investment may come much later (possibly years) than the investment.

Such analyses have also been performed at herd level as well as at regional and national level. Due to the immense herd-to-herd variation, it has often been shown that the optimum decision may vary between herds and regions.

For example, for BVDV infections, reviews of studies of 'the most optimal strategy' at herd level have favoured both a 'do nothing' strategy, and different kinds of interventions such as a 'test-and-cull' or a vaccination strategy (Houe, 2003; Saatkamp et al., 2006). The optimal strategy at herd level may depend on herd-specific conditions - in particular the risk of reintroduction of the infection and certainly also on decisions at the national level.

A situation may occur where some herds decide to live with the infection, whereas other farmers in the same area prefer to eradicate it. Such a situation, where decisions are made on a herd-to-herd basis, can be detrimental when dealing with infectious diseases due to the risk of spread of the pathogen, and it is more appropriate in this case that the decision is made at a higher level.

3.5. Change in costs and benefit over time during a control or eradication programme

The potential costs and benefits of different control strategies at the regional or national level will vary over time depending on the reduction in occurrence of infection. Fig. 3.2 illustrates the potential costs and benefits of three major 'approaches': do nothing; control; or eradication. If eradication can be achieved, the control expenditures will be low and the benefit high when reaching the monitoring phase (Fig. 3.2).

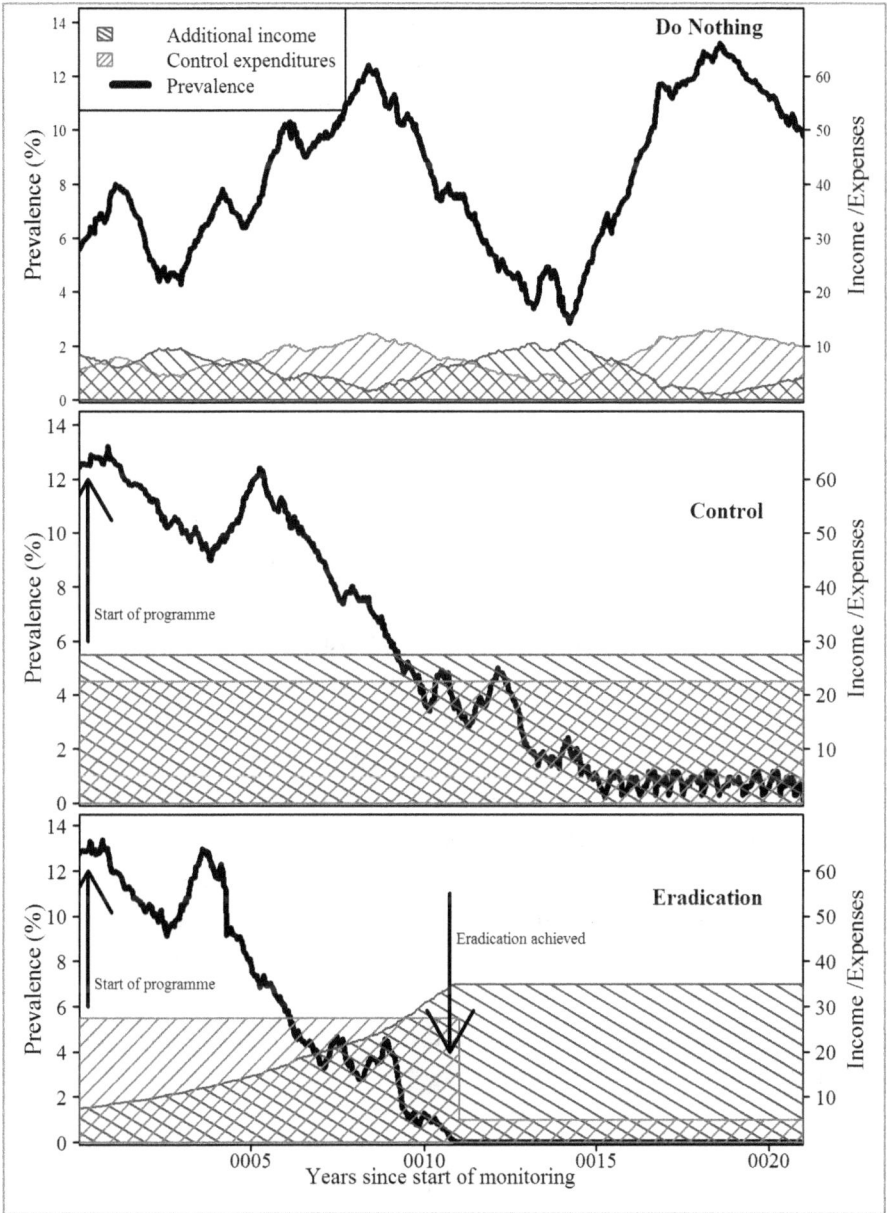

Figure 3.2. Schematic representation of potential control expenditures and additional income of three major 'strategies': do nothing; control; and eradication. The numbers on the axes are arbitrary numbers.

For endemic diseases, empirical data is often too sparse to perform a cost-benefit analysis at the national level. For BVDV infections, reviews on national eradication programmes or simulation of such programmes

19

have been shown to be cost-effective after only a few years, or over the programme period (Houe, 2003; Houe & Larsen, 2010). However, another cost-benefit analysis review at national level shows a different conclusion due to the variation of preconditions for eradication between countries (Saatkamp et al., 2006). In particular, the estimated programme costs have varied considerably from one study to another, and therefore an important element for countries having started eradication programmes is the elaboration of cost-effective test-strategies (see also Chapter 5).

3.6. Socioeconomics in a wider context

In many studies, only the direct effect on production, as well as costs for treatment and other interventions are considered. However, there can be a substantial additional effect on production economy if market prices and consumer attitudes are included. The cost-benefit analysis can be done on a wider scale to also include market prices. Thus, if disease eradication is completed, more products can be supplied for less cost and hence the market price may go down for the benefit of consumers (see e.g. Losinger, 2005 concerning MAP infections and Weldegebriel et al., 2009 on BVDV). Such a mechanism may even (at least theoretically) have the consequence that farmers who are initially free of infection may not have great interest in a programme, because they already have an efficient production. They can therefore have an economic advantage of being free of disease, while other herds in the country are infected. Therefore, it is important to stress that disease freedom in a larger area considerably reduces the risk of reinfection and therefore all farmers are anticipated to benefit from the programme in the long run.

Consumer attitudes concerning certain foodstuffs have been shown to be important if there are, for example food safety issues or problems with animal welfare, and they may therefore buy fewer products (Wells et al., 1998). This could be utilised as a strong motivator to initiate eradication programmes. Furthermore, presence of some diseases can result in limited or denied access to certain markets, and eradication of diseases in general makes it easier to export products (Rushton, 2009).

References

Bennett RM, Christiansen K, Clifton-Hadley RS, 1999. Estimating the costs associated with endemic diseases of dairy cattle. Journal of Dairy Research 66: 455–459.

Houe H, 2003. Economic impact of BVDV infections in dairies. Biologicals 31: 137-143

Houe H, Larsen LE, 2010. The impact of viral diseases on cattle production with emphasis on bovine virus diarrhoea virus. XXVI World Buiatrics congress: Updates on ruminant production and medicine, Santiago, Chile, 14-18 November 2010, 199-216.

Losinger W, 2005. Economic impact of Johne's disease on US dairy operations. Journal of Dairy Research 72: 425-432.

McInerney JP, Howe KS, Schepers JA, 1992. A framework for the economic analyses of disease in farm livestock. Preventive Veterinary Medicine 13:137–54.

Nielsen TD, Kudahl AB, Østergaard S, Nielsen LR, 2013. Gross margin losses due to *Salmonella* Dublin infection in Danish dairy cattle herds estimated by simulation modelling. Preventive Veterinary Medicine 111: 51-62.

Rushton J, 2009. The economics of animal health and production. CAB International 2009, Oxfordshire, United Kingdom.

Saatkamp HW, Stott AW, Humphrey, RW, Gunn GJ, 2006. Socioeconomic aspects of BVDV control. *In* EU Thematic Network on Control of Bovine Viral Diarrhoea Virus (BVDV), QLRT – 2001-01573: Position Paper, pp. 99-133.

Weldegebriel HT, Gunn GJ, Stott AW, 2009. Evaluation of producer and consumer benefits resulting from eradication of bovine viral diarrhoea (BVD) in Scotland, United Kingdom. Preventive Veterinary Medicine 88: 49-56.

Wells SH, SL Ott, A Hillberg Seitzinger. 1998. Key health issues for dairy cattle – new and old. Journal of Dairy Science 81: 3029-3035.

4

Biosecurity: actions to mitigate transmission of infectious diseases

4.1. Introduction

Biosecurity is an essential part of preventive veterinary medicine (i.e. preventing disease in animals and animal populations) and veterinary public health (i.e. promotion of animal and human health at sector, regional, national and international level). According to the Animal Health Strategy proposed by the European Commission in 2007, 'biosecurity refers to those measures taken to keep diseases out of populations, herds, or groups of animals where they do not currently exist or to limit the spread of disease within the herd' (Anon., 2007). This implies development of biosecurity plans at all appropriate structural levels (i.e. within-farm, between-farm, at regional and national level). According to the World Organisation for Animal Health (OIE), a biosecurity plan, 'identifies potential pathways for the introduction and spread of disease in a zone or compartment, and describes the measures which are being or will be applied to mitigate the disease risks if applicable, in accordance with the recommendations in the Terrestrial Code' (OIE, 2013). Biosecurity should not be confused with the concept of 'biosafety', which is mainly concerned with the protection of humans against potentially harmful microorganisms or biological substances, and is frequently used in laboratory settings and in prevention of bioterrorism.

Numerous research studies have underpinned the crucial importance of continuously high biosecurity standards in livestock to effectively control and eradicate diseases and infections. This chapter aims to assess at what point we have sufficient knowledge to address the question: 'How do we design systematic disease control programmes to effectively mitigate direct and indirect transmission, both on-farm and between-farms, of infectious diseases in the milk and meat-producing cattle sectors?' We realise that some of the recommendations may differ slightly in other livestock sectors. The cattle sectors are characterised by cattle-specific consumer requests and regulations for animal welfare protection that call for use of more biosecurity-challenged open housing systems. This chapter provides an insight into the biological basis of transmission routes (Section 4.2), which in turn facilitates explanations of risk factors related to the host, the agent and the environment (Section 4.3) and specifies relevant activities to improve and optimise biosecurity, i.e. how to manage and prioritise important risk factors and transmission routes in practice (Section 4.4). Unlike other biosecurity measures, vaccination is not a strategy intended to directly avoid exposure of susceptible animals and animal populations altogether. However, it is included here because when correctly used, vaccination can reduce the spread of pathogens by shortening the duration of disease or reducing the amount of shedding from infected animals. Furthermore, it often reduces susceptibility in non-infected animals leading to a diminished spread of infection in the population (Section 4.5).

4.2. The biological basis for transmission of infection

Horizontal transmission of infection can take place either directly between an infectious animal and a susceptible animal; or indirectly via the environment, for example via biological or mechanical invertebrate vectors (e.g. mosquitos, flies and ticks), and vehicles (e.g. food, water, bedding material, boots and barn equipment, and contaminated medical products). Horizontal transmission can also be airborne when pathogens are spread in droplet nuclei or dust. Hence the barn structure, flow of animals between barn sections, and hygiene of the farm environment are important factors for transmission of many pathogens. Vertical transmission implies transmission of infectious agents from the dam to the foetus in utero, or transmission of infectious agents via semen and transferred embryos. Transmission of pathogens via colostrum or by faecal contamination from dam to calf immediately after birth is sometimes referred to as 'pseudovertical'.

It is important to know the pathogenesis of the disease in order to suggest methods to control it effectively. This implies having or obtaining sufficient evidence of: the states of infection animals can undergo following exposure to the infectious agents; related clinical signs; and changed performance in production. Often these infection states are also used diagnostically (see Chapter 5). Furthermore, relevant excretion pathways from the infectious individuals, and excretion patterns (including amount of pathogens shed, duration and peak excretion time related to each of the infection states), must be determined (Fig. 4.1). These fundamental issues differ markedly between different types of infections, as illustrated in Chapter 11 for BVDV, *S.* Dublin and paratuberculosis. Furthermore, host characteristics such as age, gender, breed and immunological status can affect the probability of becoming infected, and of becoming clinically ill from the infection; the duration and severity of illness; the duration of time spent in each of the infection states; and the probability of recovery. Thus, there is much variation in the probability of infection transmission due to the determinants or risk factors related to the *host*, the *agent* or the *environment* (the classical 'host-agent-environment triad') (Fig. 4.2).

The identification of possible transmission routes, the estimation of the relative importance, and the levels of exposure caused by the identified transmission routes, are all important parts of the epidemiological investigation supporting the development of effective control programmes. Such investigations may involve direct measurements of environmental contamination and isolation of infectious agents in vectors and vehicles to identify potential exposure risks to the animals. However, because some infectious agents survive better outside the host than others, and because some multiply in vectors or vehicles whilst others do not, it may not be enough to know that the agent is present or to what degree it is present, but rather whether transmission of infection actually occurs via a given route. Therefore, observational risk-factor studies are often used to identify and evaluate the relative importance of transmission routes with significant and biologically important effects on the spread of infections (see Section 4.3).

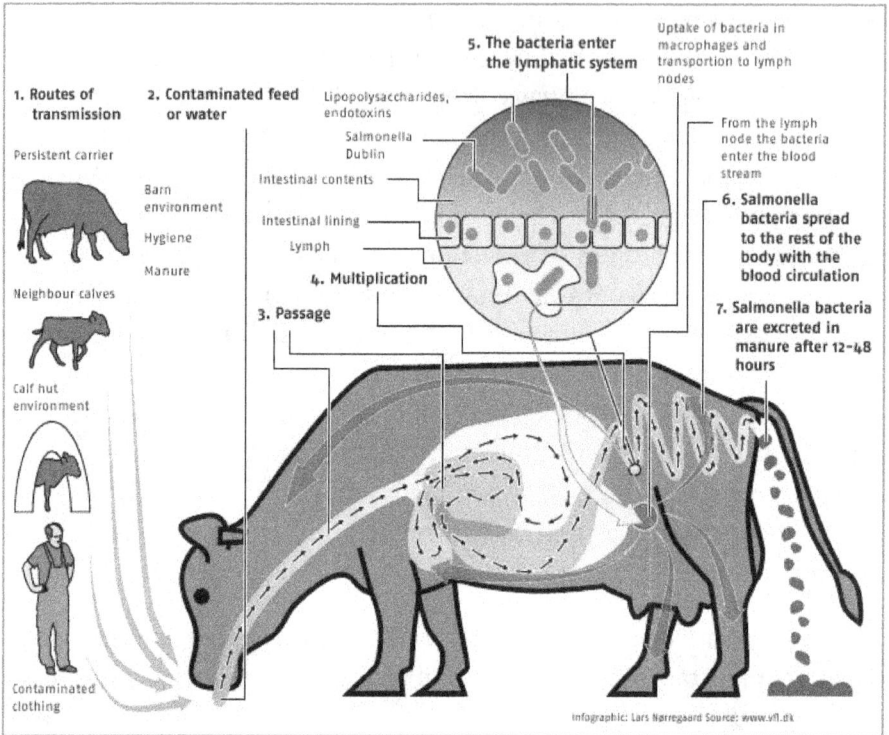

Figure 4.1. Illustration of important elements in the pathogenesis of *S.* Dublin infection in cattle to be considered when designing effective disease control programmes. (Copyright: Knowledge Centre of Agriculture, www.vfl.dk).

The characteristics of transmission of pathogens between hosts are governed by external and internal mechanisms that can be divided into: 1) exposure and entry of the host, followed by 2) invasion and dissemination, 3) different infection stages with or without excretion, 4) excretion patterns, and 5) external survival of the pathogen. Some pathogens have several different hosts with different transmission routes and infection cycles in each species, and some of these hosts can serve as reservoirs of the pathogen, ensuring the survival of the pathogen external to the primary host. These elements of transmission routes and infection cycles are essential to understanding the biological basis for transmission of infections (Figs. 4.1, 4.2 and 4.3):

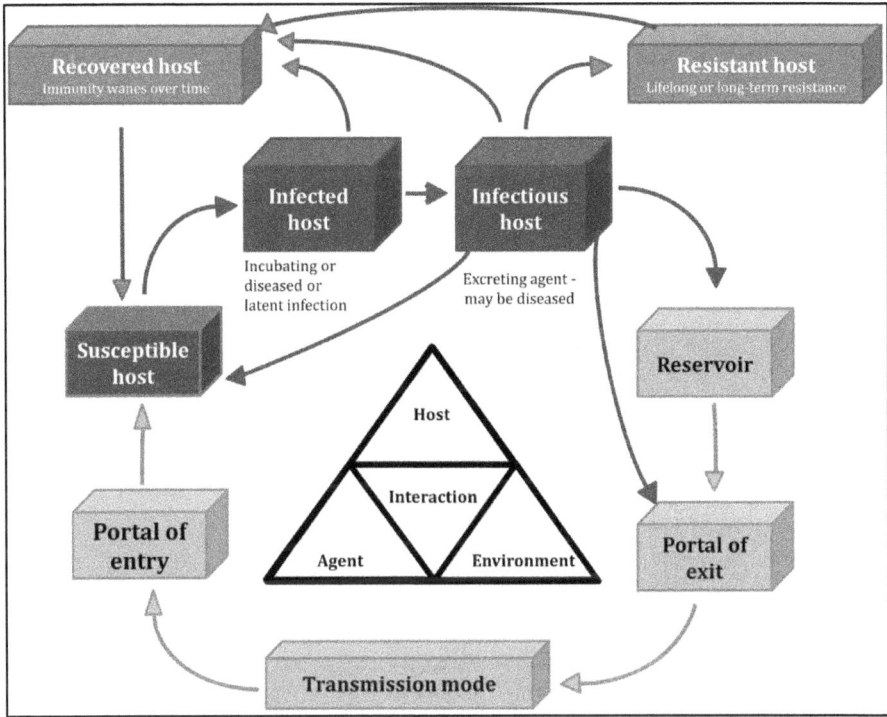

Figure 4.2. Illustration of important elements in the infection cycle and transmission of pathogens in populations.

1. **Exposure and entry routes.** When a pathogen has been physically encountered by a host, we say that the host has been *exposed*. Only if the pathogen is taken up by the host through a *portal of entry* and survives and spreads further in the host will the exposure have resulted in *entry* of the host. For example, the host may ingest infectious agents orally in contaminated feed or water, or from licking a contaminated surface or other animals. Agents may also be inhaled in droplets, dust or air that enters barns through ventilation systems, or that are spread in the barn environment during cleaning. Other entry routes of infection include the eyes, teat canal, vagina/uterus, through the skin in wounds, by insect bites or via injections with contaminated needles (iatrogenic).

2. **Invasion and dissemination.** Upon exposure, the pathogens will invade the host, disseminate, survive and multiply in many different ways depending on the exposure route(s) as well as the agent and host characteristics. For example, some enteric pathogens remain in the gut lumen upon ingestion and mainly affect the enteric environment and functions, if they are able to colonise the epithelium. Other enteric pathogens will enter the gut epithelial cells, penetrate to the underlying tissues, and spread to the blood and the lymphatic system from the entrance site, or pass to other parts of the gastrointestinal tract or other organs. Many pathogens are capable of expressing different degrees of invasion and dissemination depending on the resilience of the host. When the agent has disseminated in the host, this individual will be considered *infected*.

Infection stages. The infection cycle in an infected host varies tremendously between individuals, and different pathogens differ in the number and duration of infection stages. After uptake and entry of the pathogen, the length of time before the host starts to excrete the pathogen will vary. The period from exposure until the host begins to excrete the organism and become *infectious* is termed '*the latency period*', and we say that the host is '*latently infected*' or that it is '*a latent carrier*'. We cannot simply tell by looking at the host that it is infected, but some infected hosts will at some point start to exhibit clinical signs. The time from exposure to onset of clinical signs is '*the incubation period*'. Sometimes the latent period and the incubation period are the same. Occasionally, the host will begin to excrete the pathogen before it exhibits clinical signs, in which case the latent period is shorter than the incubation period. Conversely, sometimes the host exhibits clinical signs before excretion begins. Usually we would not consider the host latently infected, if it is showing clinical signs. Some hosts never exhibit any clinical signs, and as long as these hosts continue to be infected, we say that they are *subclinically* infected. During both the latent and infectious periods, the pathogens are present and circulating in the host, and both infection stages may affect the performance of the animal. However, performance may also be affected when the host is no longer infected, e.g. if tissue damage, weight loss or growth retardation have occurred. Fig. 4.3 illustrates different types of infections with differing orders and lengths of infection stages. It is important to distinguish between disease (illustrated above the timeline) and infectiousness (illustrated below the timeline), and to understand that these are rarely fully synchronous. For descriptions of the infection stages of BVDV, *S. Dublin* and paratuberculosis we refer to Chapter 11.

3. **Excretion patterns.** Transmission of pathogens to other hosts can begin as soon as the infected animal starts to excrete them. We say that the animal has become *infectious*. The duration and concentration of pathogens excreted depend on the *exit routes* and host characteristics such as age, immune status and whether the host is clinically affected. Sometimes pathogens can pass through specific organs without colonisation or interacting with the host in any way. We call this *passive passage*. In practice, it may be difficult (if not impossible) to separate this from true invasive infection, although pathogen-specific immune responses may in some scenarios be useful for differentiation.

4. **External survival and transmission of the pathogen.** Upon excretion, some smaller pathogens can be transmitted over longer distances, being airborne in droplet nuclei or attached to dust particles. Most commonly, however, transmission occurs directly from one individual to another by close physical contact (e.g. touching, scratching, licking or biting) or through aerosols over short distances from coughing animals. Depending on the ability of the pathogens to survive in the environment, indirect transmission can occur via intermediary involvement of another host, object or substance (reservoirs) or via aerosols created during cleaning procedures. Indirect transmission can be either vehicle-borne (e.g. food, water, bedding, equipment for handling animals, instruments, biological products, clothing, boots, contaminated medical products), or vector-borne, involving invertebrates (e.g. flies, mosquitoes, ticks etc.) carrying pathogens between vertebrate hosts. The final uptake will depend both upon the new host's susceptibility (immunity) and the infectious dose(s) to which the host is exposed (Houe et al., 2004a).

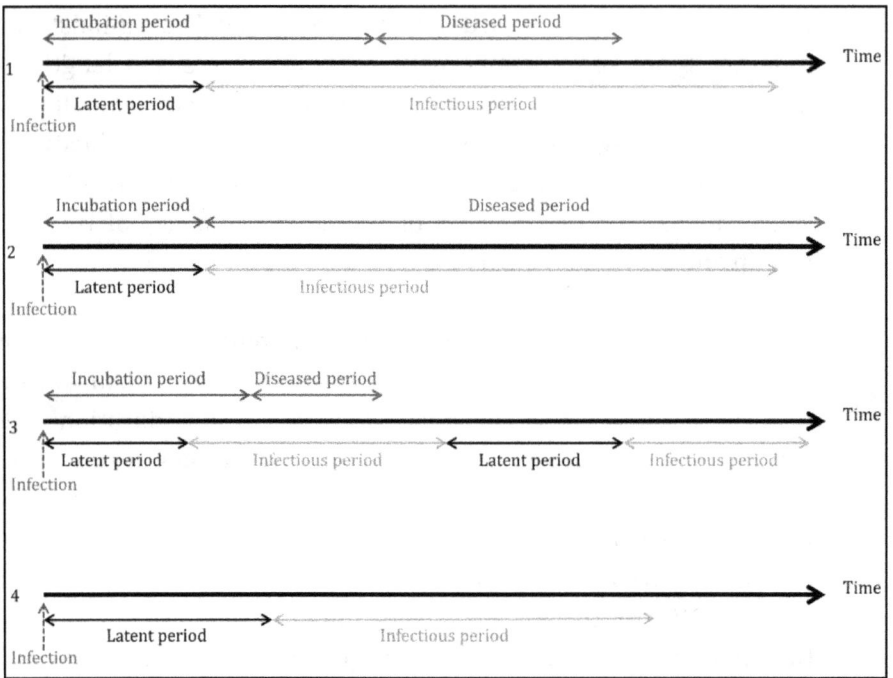

Figure 4.3. Examples of diseases with different durations of infection stages.

4.3. Risk factors for transmission of infection

The basic understanding of the infection stages and likely transmission routes provides an indication of potential risk factors for transmission, and hence relevant activities for appropriate methods and level of biosecurity, eventually leading to the control of infection spread. However, because differences in host and agent characteristics cause variation in the probability of transmission of different pathogens, risk factors must be systematically investigated in real-life situations. This will give an indication of which risk factors are most important, and which actions (i.e. procedures to ensure or enhance biosecurity) will have the highest impact on the control of the infection in question. Some biosecurity procedures are universal, meaning that they prevent the spread of many pathogens (e.g. 'all-in-all-out' barn section management with cleaning and disinfection between groups of animals). Other biosecurity procedures are effective against a specific or small group of pathogens (e.g. use of calving pens dedicated only to animals that test

30

positive for paratuberculosis, or isolation of animals with clinical signs of salmonellosis).

Host-related risk factors can include traits such as genetics, immunity, age, species and breed. For example, young animals can be very susceptible to specific agents just after they have lost the immunity that was passively transferred via colostrum. In addition vaccination, and to some extent feeding strategies can affect the susceptibility of the host and the excretion of infectious agents. The pathogens show variation in their ability to survive in the environment, enter a new host, spread within the host and be excreted again as discussed in Section 4.2, and they also vary with regard to virulence. This may lead to different levels of morbidity and mortality related to the spread of the infection, which in turn affects the infection dynamics. Finally, the environmental risk factors include a large number of variables related to the: type of production system; management and climate (e.g. housing density); cleaning procedures; transportation; temperature and humidity in the barn; and many others. These variables may result in the spread and growth of the pathogen to a level exceeding the infectious dose, resulting in infections in susceptible hosts upon exposure. The various risk factors related to the host, the agent and the environment may also interact with each other. Therefore, the transmission of infection in one population setting can be quite different to that in another. Hence, the investigations of risk factors usually involve observational studies of the relevant target populations in such a way as to allow for analysis of confounding and interacting risk factors, while also taking into account the underlying structure of the data. In analysis of livestock herds this often requires taking into account so-called hierarchical structures, i.e. animals clustered within the same herd are more alike (or correlated) than animals between different herds. Risk factors are often determined as those that lead to increased (or decreased) risk of transmission of pathogens between herds, and those that lead to increased (or decreased) risk of transmission within herds. Risk factors that decrease the risk of transmission are preventive and are equally as important to identify. In many cases, the interpretation of the effect of a risk factor relies on the way it was measured and analysed in the study, so this needs to be carefully considered when planning and reporting the study. It is therefore strongly recommended to adhere to state-of-the-art epidemiological methods in the pursuit of evidence to support disease control programmes (Dohoo et al., 2009; Houe et al., 2004b).

4.4. The implementation of biosecurity procedures

When appropriate risk-factor studies have been performed and the most essential transmission routes have been identified, the next step is to implement procedures that enhance biosecurity in the population of interest. This may be done at different levels and encouraged both centrally (e.g. through legislation, sector policies and standards including own-check programmes where each producer has to document that he/she complies with certain production standards), and locally (e.g. decided by the owner or manager of the herd and implemented by all employees). It is well recognised that obtaining an adequate biosecurity level can be challenging in livestock populations, especially in large cattle herds where the hygiene level, population size and contact between groups of animals are important risk factors for transmission of pathogens (Nielsen et al., 2012). Several studies have been performed to investigate constraints to the implementation of biosecurity procedures, including farmers' perception and willingness to invest in biosecurity; and the role and perceptions of veterinary practitioners, auxiliary industries and policy makers (Ellis-Iversen et al., 2010; Gunn et al., 2008; Kristensen and Jakobsen, 2011; Toma et al., 2013). Frequently, certain stakeholders perceive the responsibility of biosecurity as 'somebody else's problem', and may give up without ever having tried to implement the most obviously effective biosecurity procedures, such as restrictive trade policy, avoiding mingling of livestock from different farms, appropriate flow of animals in the herd, barn sectioning and systematic cleaning procedures. Perceptions such as, 'if my neighbour does not do the same, it is not worth it' are common. Hence, the perception of responsibility and feasibility often becomes a major obstacle in disease control programmes. It is therefore crucial to direct sufficient attention to how to solve these issues in order to ensure success in the programme. Motivation, proof of concept and communication are all essential when attempting to improve the stakeholder's perceptions of, and compliance with the overall aim of the programme. We refer to Chapters 3, 6, 9 and 11 for more information and inspiration about these elements in disease control programmes for endemic diseases.

A full list of possible biosecurity measures and procedures would be long and diverse, and the imagination alone can put a limit on the actions that can be taken to improve biosecurity. Therefore, only some are mentioned here. Biosecurity procedures may include administrative measures that apply to all, such as test certificates (either paper-based or electronic/online) required to move animals between herds; mandatory quarantine of imported animals; prevention or restriction of movement of animals between herds with different disease statuses; and regulation of contact between different regions or herds with specific characteristics ('compartments', e.g. herds allowing outdoor housing vs. strictly indoor housing). Most of the administrative biosecurity measures are directed towards prevention of transmission of infections into the country and between herds. Sector-wise, own-check programmes frequently include biosecurity checks. Some of these may be governed by national legislation (e.g. animal density and pen size requirements) whereas others are governed by the sectors' own quality standards (e.g. tidy barn environment, rodent and insect control, and cleanliness of animals). The biosecurity standards determined at sector level aim to prevent infections being spread both between herds, between animals, and to food products being produced in the herd (e.g. milk and meat). These frequently attempt to protect animal health, animal welfare and public health simultaneously. Finally, many biosecurity procedures are planned and decided locally at farm level (e.g. purchase policies; the feeding and management of different age groups; calving management and hygiene of calving pens and calf housing facilities; change of clothes between barns; use of boot washing and disinfection facilities between barn sections; and cleaning of feeding tables and drinking troughs). The choice of cleaning procedures, detergents and disinfectants is determined by a combination of the materials in the environment and the infectious agents being targeted. The availability of the products and the legislation concerning chemicals used in detergents and disinfectants continually change. Hence, it is recommended to seek professional advice for given situations requiring new or adjusted cleaning procedures in livestock herds.

Box 4.1. List of biosecurity procedures in cattle farms, not in order of priority (adapted from Moore et al. 2008)

Perform risk assessment

Follow biosecurity plan

On-farm biosecurity signage

Employee training

Restrictive purchase / closed herd policy

Avoid mingling with animals from other farms, e.g. at shows or on pasture

Perimeter fence, locked gates and doors

Appropriate animal flow including not moving older animals back in the system

Animal identification and record-keeping of location and health status of animals

Disease awareness, isolation of sick animals, and culling protocols

Calving management, e.g. clean calving pen, separate cows at calving/single calving pens, remove calf immediately after calving

Colostrum management

Young stock (YS) management and housing

Manure storage and management

Vector control (i.e. rodents, insects, birds, pets, wild life)

Methods to prevent feed and water contamination

Cleaning routines for feeding tables and water troughs

Equipment and tool cleaning and disinfection

Do not share equipment / tools between barn sections

Clean clothing and hand sanitation

Footbaths or disposable boots

Control of visitor and vehicle access, disinfection of vehicles

Quarantine or isolation of animals entering or returning to the farm

Appropriate pick up and disposal of dead stock

Vaccination if feasible and effective

Maintenance of visitor logs (rarely used in cattle herds)

Shower-in procedures (rarely used in cattle herds)

Employee or owner restrictions on owning livestock (rarely used in cattle herds)

Specific biosecurity procedures that have been reportedly used in production animal farms include the long list shown in Box 4.1, however other procedures may be relevant for individual farms (Sarrazin et al., 2014). It is important that the practical implementation is specified clearly for each farm so that all employees are able to comply with the biosecurity plan (Moore et al., 2008).

4.5. Vaccination

As mentioned at the beginning of the chapter, vaccination is not an avoidance strategy (setting it apart from other biosecurity measures), but rather in most cases, a way to improve the effect of a control programme by lowering the susceptibility of previously unexposed animals and reducing the excretion of infectious agents from those that become infected. Use of vaccination is only recommended if effective vaccines are available. Yet even if effective vaccines are available, it may not be cost-effective to use them in a control or eradication programme. Economic analyses are required to clarify the cost-benefits of using vaccination as opposed to relying on other disease control methods. Vaccination can rarely stand alone as a means to eradicate infections from a cattle population. Nonetheless, at the initiative of the Food and Agriculture Organisation (FAO) and OIE in 1994, the viral cattle infection rinderpest ('cattle plague') was eradicated globally through a combination of an effective vaccine and surveillance, and in 2011 OIE declared the world free from rinderpest. This was possible due to the direct transmission routes of the virus between individual cattle, and its poor survival in the environment; combined with the availability of an effective vaccine, which rendered vaccinated animals essentially non-susceptible and preventing excretion of the agent. With many other infectious agents, it is a lot more complicated to eliminate all of the important transmission routes, and in some cases the vaccine strain may even be shed into the environment. Furthermore, effective vaccines do not exist for every important pathogen in livestock. Therefore, good biosecurity remains an essential element of all disease control programmes, and must be an essential element in the daily management of livestock herds, not just during a herd health crisis or during a regional or national outbreak of disease.

References

Anon., 2007. A new Animal Health Strategy for the European Union (2007-2013) where 'Prevention is better than cure'. The EU Commission COM 539 (2007).

Dohoo I, Martin W, Stryhn H, 2009. Veterinary Epidemiologic Research. VER Inc., Charlottetown, Prince Edwards Island, Canada.

Ellis-Iversen JE, Cook AJ, Watson E, Nielen M, Larkin L, Wooldridge M, Hogeveen H, 2010. Perceptions, circumstances and motivators that influence implementation of zoonotic control programs on cattle farms. Preventive Veterinary Medicine 93: 276-285.

Gunn GJ, Heffernan C, Hall M, McLeod A, Hovi M, 2008. Measuring and comparing constraints to improved biosecurity amongst GB farmers, veterinarians and the auxiliary industries. Preventive Veterinary Medicine 84: 310-323.

Houe H, Ersbøll AK, Nielsen LR, 2004a. Nature of data. In: Houe H, Ersbøll AK, Toft N (Eds): Introduction to Veterinary Epidemiology, 2004. Biofolia, Frederiksberg C, Denmark.

Houe H, Ersbøll AK, Toft N, 2004b. Introduction to Veterinary Epidemiology. Biofolia, Frederiksberg C, Denmark.

Kristensen E, Jakobsen EB, 2011. Danish dairy farmers' perception of biosecurity. Preventive Veterinary Medicine 99: 122-129.

Moore DA, Merryman ML, Hartman ML, Klingborg DJ, 2008. Comparison of published recommendations regarding biosecurity practices for various production animal species and classes. Journal of American Veterinary Medical Association 233: 249-56.

Nielsen LR, Kudahl AB, Østergaard S, 2012. Age-structured dynamic, stochastic and mechanistic simulation model of *Salmonella* Dublin infection within dairy herds. Preventive Veterinary Medicine 105: 59-74.

OIE, 2013. Glossary of the OIE Terrestrial Animal Health Code http://www.oie.int/fileadmin/Home/eng/Health_standards/tahc/2010

/en_glossaire.htm#terme_plan_de_securite_biologique (accessed 5 June 2013).

Sarrazin S, Cay AB, Laureyns J, Dewulf J, 2014. A survey on biosecurity and management practices in selected Belgian cattle farms. Preventive Veterinary Medicine. http://dx.doi.org/10.1016/j.prevetmed.2014.07.014

Toma L, Stott AW, Heffernan C, Ringrose S, Gunn GJ, 2013. Determinants of biosecurity behaviour of British cattle and sheep farmers - a behavioural economics analysis. Preventive Veterinary Medicine 108: 321-333.

5

Establishment of purpose-specific and systematic test-strategies

5.1. Introduction

Historically, national eradication of infections has been achieved without access to any diagnostic tests, and even without knowing the pathogen. This was the case with the early efforts against rinderpest, where rigorous biosecurity measures and elimination of diseased animals were sufficient for its eradication from Denmark in 1782 (OIE, 2013). However for many infectious agents, identification of both diseased and non-diseased subclinically infected animals may be crucial for control of the specific agent.

This chapter describes the considerations necessary to establish test-strategies of relevance for specific purposes ('fit for purpose') at the animal, herd, regional, or national level. Any systematic test and elimination strategy at the animal, herd or regional/national population level must take into account these purposes, together with the available diagnostic tests for the specific infection. Specific applications of BVDV, paratuberculosis and *S.* Dublin are described in Chapter 11, while the terminology introduced here is illustrated using examples at the end of this chapter. Some minor examples are also given within the text.

5.2. Elements of a test-strategy

The overall aim of establishing a test-strategy is to create a decision-support system to optimise the use of resources available for the overall purpose, which in this context is control or eradication of the infection. In a control programme that is not necessarily aiming at eradicating the infection (see Chapter 3), it might be beneficial to reduce the prevalence to a target level and keep it below this level. Multiple test-strategies can be of relevance in the different phases of the programme and even within the same phase. For example, identification and containment of infectious animals may be of primary importance in the control phase, whereas identification of newly infected herds is often a priority during surveillance in disease-free or low-prevalence populations. In addition, surveillance of beef cattle and dairy cattle may be different in the same phase due to differences in production and management aspects, e.g. beef cattle will typically not produce milk and thus cannot provide samples for individual or bulk tank milk (BTM) testing.

Specification of a test-strategy for specific pathogens should include:

a) the purpose(s) and objectives that testing should fulfil, including a specification of the target population;
b) the interpretation of a positive or a negative test-result; and
c) the decisions and actions that given test-results will support.

5.3. Purposes of testing

A test-strategy should be 'fit-for-purpose' (OIE, 2003), preferably with specific emphasis on the overall purpose of the programme. Specific purposes of diagnostic testing could be:

- **to increase animal welfare or herd profitability** via identification and subsequent management of diseased or affected animals, e.g. detection of animals clinically affected by the infectious agent, or animals that have reduced productivity due to being infected (Example 5.1);
- **to increase food safety** via identification and management of affected animals or herds which may expose humans to the infectious agent (Example 5.2);
- **to reduce transmission of the pathogen** through identification and containment of infectious animals, e.g. detection and removal of animals which spread pathogens in sufficient quantities to allow infection to be transmitted to a susceptible animal either directly or via the environment (Examples 5.1, 5.2 and 5.3).

These purposes may state specific tasks to decision makers, but may also require description of additional specific objectives, for example:

- **to classify herds as infected** (Example 5.2);
- **to monitor infection** via identification of infected animals, e.g. detecting animals hosting the infectious agent without necessarily being diseased or infectious themselves (Example 5.3);
- **to monitor clearance of infection**, e.g. detect animals that have cleared the infection and are resistant, or are recovered and returning to the susceptible infection state (Example 5.4);
- **to certify animals or herds free (or at low risk) of infection**, both at individual and at herd level (Example 5.4);
- **to discriminate between vaccinated and infected animals**.

Programmes targeting the various infectious agents may not include all these purposes, and conversely the list may not be complete for all infections. For each infectious agent, each programme and each phase of the programme, it is important to establish the relevant testing purpose(s). Since there may be several purposes in one programme, and since the same test can be used for multiple purposes in different test-strategies, the same test-result can lead to different actions. It is important for this to be clear in the information strategy of the programme, as it tends to create confusion amongst farmers and other decision makers. (See Chapter 9 for more details on information and education strategies.)

5.4. Interpretation of test-results
5.4.1. Target conditions

Once the purpose is known, a test-strategy can be devised. Knowledge of the pathogenesis is required to establish the 'target conditions', which are relevant to a specific purpose and thus a specific test-strategy. The target condition is to be decided upon, and may be on different levels: the animal, the herd, the region etc. We may not be able to detect this particular condition with the available diagnostic tests, but the ultimate aim of the test-strategy is to closely target this condition.

Target conditions could include:

a) 'diseased animals', because we are interested only in having healthy animals for ethical as well as for economic reasons. Animals with reduced production due to the infectious agent are considered 'diseased' or 'affected';

b) 'infectious animals', because these are responsible for transmitting the infectious agent in the present state, regardless of whether or not they are showing signs of disease;

c) 'infected animals', because they are at risk of becoming infectious or diseased in the future;

d) 'recovered animals' or 'infected and recovered animals', because they are indicators of previous exposure to the pathogen; or

e) 'animals constituting a risk of human exposure' to the infectious agent, because the agent is in tissues intended for human consumption.

Additional target conditions may be of relevance for some infectious agents, but not all conditions listed are of relevance to all agents. For example, target condition e) may only be considered relevant for zoonotic agents, unless it is considered unethical to expose humans to animals harbouring the agent. For example, BVDV is not zoonotic, but some people may not wish to consume BVD infected animals. Other pathogens may not be a risk to human health, but may still be undesirable in meat or milk for aesthetic or quality assurance reasons. Some agents may have an unknown zoonotic potential and consequently the precautionary principle should prevail.

If knowledge about the pathogenesis is not sufficient to describe specific targets, this knowledge has to be established with some level of certainty before appropriate test-strategies can be developed. Yet determining the desired condition for detection is the first step towards detecting it and thus gaining further knowledge. After the target condition has been established, it is first necessary to establish a case definition before the condition can be detected (Fig. 5.1).

Purpose	→	Target condition	→	Case definition

— reduce transmission → — Infectious → — 1bacterium detected
(identification and isolation   animals   (in faecal sample of 3g)
of infectious animals)

— increase welfare → — animals in → — animals with
(identification of   pain   diarrhoea
diseased animals)

— to monitor infection → — infected → — animals w. pathology
(identification of   animals   (where ≥1/20 tissues from xx
infected animals)   organs resulted in finding of yy)

— safeguard food → — animals with → — animals w. bacteria
(identification of   bacteraemia   (from ≥1 of 10 muscle
animals with bacteraemia)

— to .... — animals .... — animals ....

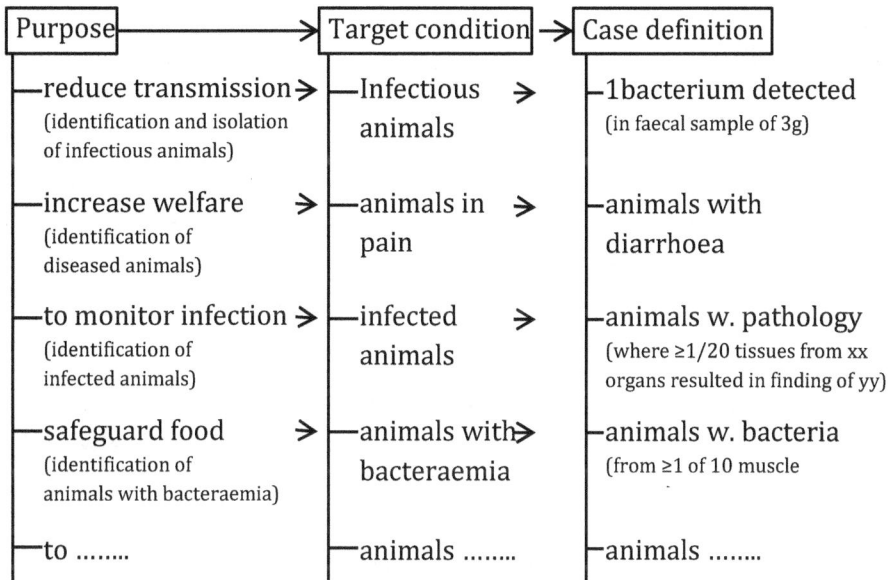

Figure 5.1. Relationship between purpose, target condition and case definition including various examples.

5.4.2. Case definitions

A practical realisation of a target condition is the 'case definition' (Fig. 5.2). In many epidemiology texts, it is referred to as a 'reference standard' or a 'gold standard'. The latter is a misnomer and should be avoided (Wilks, 2001). A good case definition is closely related to the target condition that it describes. For example, a case definition for a persistently BVDV infected animal may include: i) detection of BVDV virus in the buffy coat of a blood sample, and ii) lack of BVD-specific antibodies in a serum sample from the same animal, where samples have been collected two times, approximately 3 weeks apart. In this particular example, there are several specific requirements to fulfil. If these are not all fulfilled, it is not a case and should not be considered a persistently BVD infected animal.

Not all definitions are as straightforward. For instance, a case definition for the target condition of 'MAP infectious animal' could be detection of MAP in faeces. However, if the infectious agent is present in very low quantities in faeces, the animal may not excrete enough of it to be infectious, and therefore does not meet the criteria for the target condition. Consequently, a better case definition may specify the level of MAP that should be present if the faeces should indeed be infectious to a susceptible animal. This issue may become increasingly important for many infectious agents, as diagnostic tests are developed with higher and higher analytical sensitivity. Detecting one colony forming unit (CFU) of bacteria, or traces of DNA material from an agent may not necessarily mean that this animal is an infectious case, and we would have to deal with this aspect when using the case definition or interpreting test-results.

Case definitions can be useful for test evaluations to establish a proxy for the 'true infection or disease status'. However, it may not always be feasible to determine this status in the operational phase, because the test used as 'reference standard' is too expensive or impractical to perform. Moreover, the target condition of interest is, in practice, often impossible to detect accurately. For instance, cattle can be infected with *S.* Dublin or MAP without showing clinical signs or without testing positive in any available test procedure. A *S.* Dublin or MAP infected animal may have viable bacteria in tissues or cells that would not be detected even after a very thorough necropsy followed by histology and culture of many tissue samples. We could sample numerous tissues throughout the whole carcass and may still miss the bacteria. For example, Whitlock et al. (1996) suggested sampling and culturing up to 100 tissues from cattle to determine their true MAP infection status. This would, in most cases, be very expensive and perhaps even impossible to do in practice. Therefore, we often use less costly diagnostic tests or test procedures to infer whether the animal is a case or not. It should be noted that case definitions may not always be required in the course of a programme, yet are often necessary in test evaluations.

5.4.3. The diagnostic test

The diagnostic test is usually not perfect, but we can assess the sensitivity (Se) and specificity (Sp) to determine how close they are to the target condition. For example, this can be done relative to a reference standard, or by other means (Nielsen et al., 2011). It is always preferable to use the target condition but, as mentioned, we may need to use the case definition in practice. However, the case definition is not always required, e.g. if latent class methodology is used. Ultimately, the goal is to characterise the test relative to the target condition, not the case definition, although we may have to use the latter (Fig. 5.2).

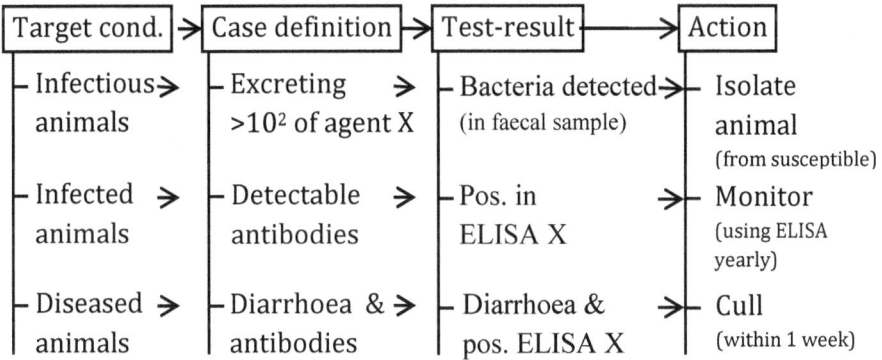

Target cond. →	Case definition →	Test-result ⟶	Action
– Infectious→ animals	– Excreting → >10² of agent X	– Bacteria detected→ (in faecal sample)	– Isolate animal (from susceptible)
– Infected → animals	– Detectable → antibodies	– Pos. in ELISA X	→– Monitor (using ELISA yearly)
– Diseased → animals	– Diarrhoea & → antibodies	– Diarrhoea & pos. ELISA X	→– Cull (within 1 week)

Figure 5.2. Relations between target condition, case definition, test-result and planned actions with various examples.

The Se expresses the probability that a subject (i.e. animal or herd) with the target condition is classified as test-positive when the test is applied to it. The Sp is the probability that animals or herds without the target condition become classified as test-negative by the test or test procedure. Note that the distinction here is 'with' or 'without' the target condition. The Se and Sp will thus differ between target conditions, even for the same test or test procedure.

The Se and Sp give information about the specific test used for a specific target condition. However, the decision maker is provided with a test-result. The predictive value of this result is of greater practical value to him/her than the Se and Sp per se, in the situation where a decision is required about an animal or a herd. The two relevant parameters are known as the positive predictive value and the negative predictive value (Nielsen et al., 2004). The former expresses the probability that a positive test-result is indeed from an animal (or herd) with the target condition, whereas the latter expresses the probability that a test-negative animal (or a herd) is from an animal (herd) without the target condition. A disadvantage of using the positive predictive value and negative predictive value is that they are dependent on the prevalence in the population and consequently may differ between populations.

Therefore, reporting of the Se and Sp is standard, but these should be converted to predictive values in specific populations in order for relevant decisions to be made. Furthermore, the predictive values may have to be adjusted during a control programme, if the prevalence changes over time (Warnick et al., 2006). Fig. 5.3 provides an example where the predictive values vary with both prevalence and age of the animals. The latter is due to increased Se with increasing age. In this example, almost perfect negative predictive values can be achieved at low prevalences, while high prevalences yield high positive predictive values.

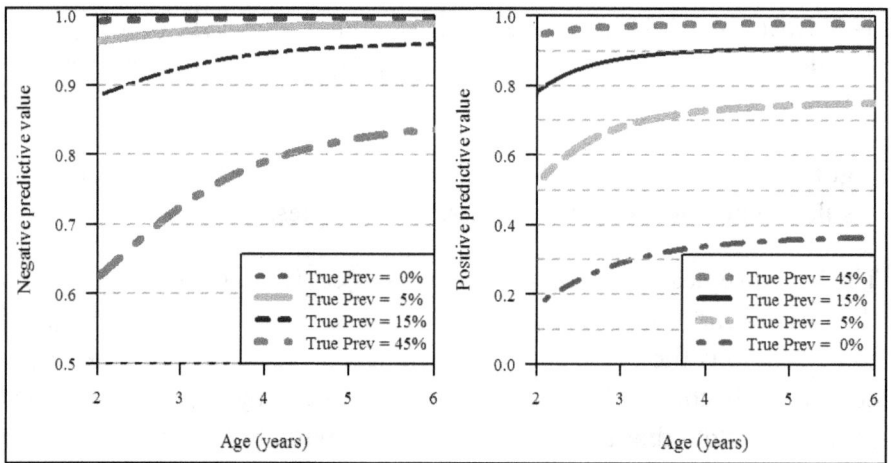

Figure 5.3. Negative (left) and positive (right) predictive values varying with both age and true prevalence (TP). The example is based on antibody ELISA for MAP, based on Sp and age-specific Se given in Nielsen et al. (2013). Negative predictive values are particularly low at high prevalences, but almost perfect at low prevalences, whereas the opposite is the case for the positive predictive values. Age plays the biggest role for young cattle.

5.5. Decision making and action taking

The diagnostic test-results should ultimately be used for decision-making, based on the individual test-result or an aggregation of results, e.g. an apparent prevalence. A test-result not used for decision-making can be considered wasted resources, although a decision to do nothing may be practical. Decisions and actions associated with the test-result should be closely related to the purpose of testing (Fig. 5.2).

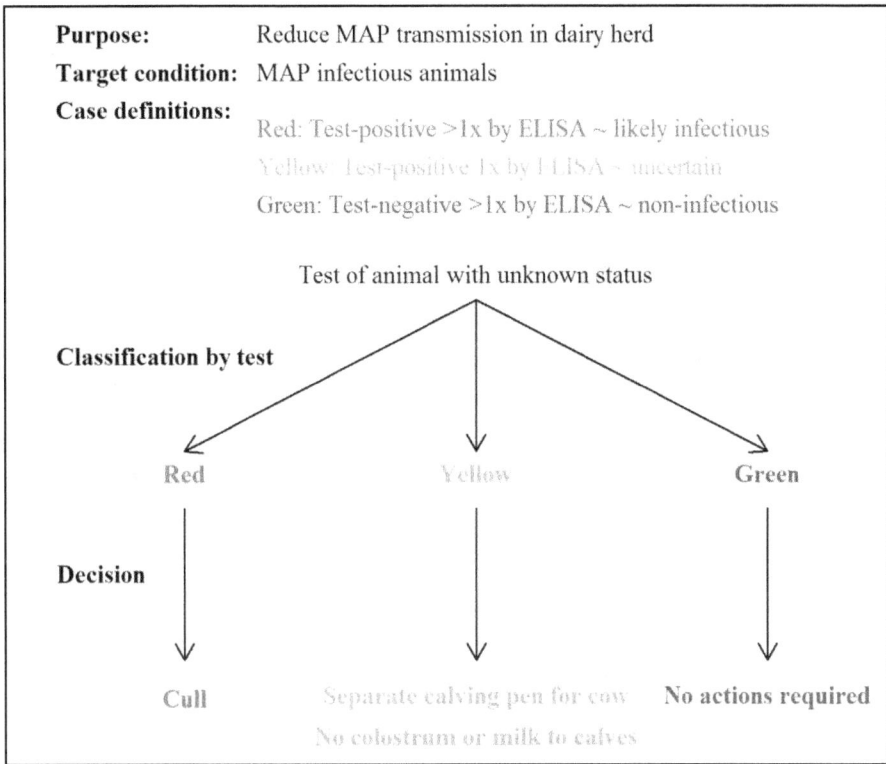

Figure 5.4. Decision diagram used for decisions following repeated testing using ELISA in the risk-based Danish MAP control programme. Samples are collected repeatedly and tested for antibodies, resulting in multiple test-results. Cows are subsequently classified based on the presumed infectious status, and actions are defined for each of these statuses. The colour codes 'red', 'yellow' and 'green' communicate three levels of risk, which can be further quantified for the decision maker, although this is not necessary.

Common actions following test-results are:

- doing nothing, e.g. if an animal is not deemed to be diseased, it should not be treated (or managed differently);
- retesting to confirm the target condition;
- isolation or culling of the animal/herd to avoid transmission to other susceptible animals/herds;

- appropriate slaughtering circumstances for test-positive animals or herds with high prevalence to avoid contamination of meat products for human consumption.

Decision diagrams can be useful to draw specific attention to the recommended actions following test-results of a specific test-strategy. Fig. 5.4 provides an example used for reducing transmission of MAP in the Danish MAP control programme (Nielsen, 2007).

5.6. Aggregation of test information

Several population levels may be of interest, and should be defined in the purpose of testing, for example the test should provide information about an animal, a herd, or perhaps a region. Aggregation of test information should therefore be considered. Aggregation can be based on the sample (e.g. mixing milk from individual cows into a bulk tank and then sample from there) or based on summarising results of samples from multiple sites or animals. Se and Sp can often be calculated at each level using appropriate techniques and thus summarise such information (Christensen and Gardner, 2000). Furthermore, advanced methods are available to estimate the Se and Sp of diagnostic tests or test procedures, TP of infection, and probability of freedom from infection between and within tested herds in a population with unknown infection status (Nielsen et al, 2011). However, the main difference between Se and Sp at the animal and herd level is the level about which the test can be used to make inference. This should correspond to the purpose of testing. Example 5.4 illustrates how information from several animals was aggregated to provide information about the herd.

A test-strategy on national, regional or any lower level may include more general descriptions of the purpose, the interpretation and possible decisions following testing, but they do not differ greatly from the lower-level strategy specifications.

5.7. Combining the elements of a test-strategy

Identification of the purpose of testing, target condition and case definition, as well as considerations of how the diagnostic test should be used is pivotal to establishing a test-strategy (see Examples 5.1-5.4). Once established, the Se and Sp of the test can be determined for the relevant target conditions, and further work can be done to establish the predictive values and establish decision support diagrams. However, the setting in which tests should be used must also be considered. The setting includes considerations on the level of testing, the population of interest, the sampling material, costs of testing and logistics etc. It is important to note that sample size and frequency of testing are also relevant. They too are related to the purpose of testing, but can only be established based on knowledge of the pathogenesis and infection dynamics. For example, *S.* Dublin and BVDV infections are often transmitted to many other animals within an age cohort (see Example 5.4 on BVDV). Consequently, if we only need to determine whether or not a cohort has been exposed, it is not necessary to test all the animals. Since detection of a single or small number of infected animals would provide us with the relevant information, it is sufficient to test only an appropriate sample. However, whole-herd testing may be required to interpret the occurrence of MAP in a herd, simply because the combination of the test's low Se and an expected low prevalence will result in very few test-positive animals in many herds (Sergeant et al., 2008). Therefore, a test-strategy for one purpose related to an infection may not be useful in the case of another infection, even with the same purpose.

Sample materials also play an important role. It may be that culture of jejunal tissue samples provides high Se, but obtaining this sample material antemortem is often not feasible. Blood or faecal sampling also requires that animals are caught and managed during sampling. This can be a time-consuming process, and many farmers are reluctant to tie their animals, as they may fear long-term production losses due to handling stress, lack of access to food and water while in headlocks etc. Some cattle are kept outdoors, complicating blood or faecal sampling even further. Milk samples are often collected routinely during milk recordings, and can be a good resource in dairy herds. However, leftover milk in milking equipment may result in false-positive test-results (Mahmmod et al., 2013), and such possible adverse effects should be weighed against the ease of sampling. Options for shipment of samples to laboratories, capacity of the laboratories to test the samples and proper provision of results to the decision makers are also elements that need to be considered in the test-strategy.

The principles in the construction of a test-strategy thus include:

a) identification of the purpose of testing;
b) identification (and evaluation) of one or more tests to fulfil this purpose;
c) establishment of logistics for sampling and management of results;
d) reporting of results with specific sets of recommendations for the use of the results;
e) use of the results by the decision maker.

5.8. Summary remarks

The demands on the diagnostic test performance depend on the situation in which they are used. As already mentioned in the section on biosecurity (Chapter 4), an important purpose of testing individual animals is being able to issue test certificates. In this situation, a high Se (high negative predictive value) will be important. However, if the individual test is to be used for herd classification, where the herd Se can be increased by testing a higher number of animals, the demands on the Se may be lower. Nonetheless, tests with low Se or Sp related to one target condition may have a high Se and Sp in relation to another target condition and purpose. Therefore, the purpose and test-strategy must go hand-in-hand. In any case, the performance of the individual tests has a huge impact on the cost of the programme, and it is therefore important that the test performs as well as possible, and that the Se and Sp of the individual diagnostic tests are known. Finally, it is important to note that unused test-results are a waste of resources.

5.9. Examples

Example 5.1. Purposes, target condition, case definition, test-result and action for the BVDV transiently-infected animal with known time of infection.

BVDV infected animals can be infected in two very distinct ways: either as transiently or persistently infected (PI) (Chapter 11). The transiently-infected animal is particularly interesting as it is possible to establish the time of infection, which may indicate recent introduction of BVDV to the herd, or that an active source of transmission is present in the herd. In addition, it is possible to predict possible sequelae to the cow and the herd if the time of infection can be established.

As a result, a cow with a transient infection of known length is an obvious target condition. This can serve the purpose of 'detective follow up' (Purpose 1a) where an unknown infection source needs to be identified (e.g. transmission over the fence to cows on pasture or birth of a PI animal in the herd), or reducing future losses (Purpose 1b) due to, for example, abortion, and finally reducing future transmission (Purpose 1c) by preventing the transiently-infected cow from giving birth to a PI animal in the future. A suitable case definition is an animal changing from antibody negative to positive on blood samples taken 2-3 weeks apart (seroconverting) or showing at least a fourfold rise in antibody titre.

Depending on the purpose, different actions may be appropriate (but note that one purpose does not exclude another). For the purpose of detective follow up, the action could be to investigate if neighbour herds with animals on nearby pastures have positive infection states, or if there have been any weak calves born recently, potentially indicating the birth of PI animals which could be tested. For the purpose of preventing sequelae such as abortions or further births of PI animals, the action could be to cull the transiently-infected cow. This example illustrates that the same target condition (case definition and test-result) can serve very different purposes and hence be associated with different actions.

Purpose	Target condition	Case definition	Test-result	Action /decision
Detect source of transmission (1a and 1c)	Recent infection of immune-competent animal	Sero-conversion	Two tests 2-3 weeks apart: ELISA-Neg =>ELISA-Pos	Check neighbours Test new-born
Prevent sequelae: Abortions (1b)			Or rise in titre	Culling of cow

Example 5.2. Surveillance of *S.* Dublin dairy herd infection status based on antibody measurements on BTM samples.

S. Dublin is a bacterial gastrointestinal infection that causes disease (diarrhoea, pneumonia, septicaemia, abortions and ill-thrift), increased mortality, and production losses in infected cattle herds. Furthermore, it is an infrequent but severe invasive zoonotic infection in humans, who most frequently become infected via contaminated raw or undercooked beef, unpasteurised milk products, or direct contact to infected cattle or manure. Since animal-level testing does not provide accurate distinction between infected, infectious and non-infected cattle, surveillance and control programmes for *S.* Dublin in cattle populations are typically based on herd classifications and associated trade-restricting regulations supported by biosecurity measures in infected herds aiming to control the within-herd spread of infection (Chapter 11).

Antibody measurements (ELISA) on BTM provide a cost-effective tool for classification of dairy herds. Since single BTM test-results are too uncertain for herd classification, interpretation of the test-results usually involves assessment of a series of test-results over an extended period. The Danish dairy herd classification system is based on four consecutive BTM samples collected every 4 months and tested for level (optical density corrected ODC%) of antibodies directed against *Salmonella* serogroup D-antigens in the ELISA. If the average of the four test-results is 25 ODC% or higher the herd is classified as most likely infected with *S.* Dublin. Otherwise the herd will be classified as most likely not infected with *S.* Dublin and hence is considered a low-risk herd from which to purchase cattle for replacements or expansion of dairy herds.

The purpose of testing BTM in the surveillance and control programme for *S.* Dublin in Denmark has therefore been to reduce between-herd transmission through classification of herds into high and low risk of infection, and to provide a tool for farmers to protect their herds when purchase or alternative types of contact to other cattle herds were necessary (e.g. common grassing and participation in animal shows). The ultimate goal, however, is to increase food safety.

Purpose	Target condition	Case definition	Test-result	Action/ decision
Reduce transmission between herds	Infected herds	Herds with antibody positive animals	Mean BTM ELISA > 25 ODC%	Trade restrictions

Example 5.3. Purpose, target condition, case definition, test-result and action for animals persistently infected with BVDV.

Among the most distinctive features of BVDV infections is the foetal infection in early pregnancy followed by immune tolerance and lifelong persistent infection. The persistent infection has several consequences, including a high risk of ill-thrift and early death of the animal itself, due to mucosal disease. Additionally, the persistent infection results in a very high excretion of virus, and almost all animals in the vicinity (e.g. in the same building) will be infected within a few weeks. The pathogenesis of the persistent infection also means that no matter what the age of the animal when the persistent infection is detected, the calendar time of the foetal infection can be identified as being within a 3-4 month window. Therefore, the identification of such animals can serve several purposes, including improved welfare, economy, and reduced transmission providing this animal is slaughtered prior to developing mucosal disease.

The target condition is defined as animals that are born immunotolerant and thus PI for life. The case definition is animals in which BVDV has been detected in two samples obtained at least 3 weeks apart. There are different possibilities for the actual testing procedure; two blood samples can be collected, but in recent years ear notches have been shown to be suitable specimen as they avoid interference with colostral antibodies (Cornish et al., 2005).

The actions taken are directly linked to the purpose, i.e. slaughter the animal to prevent later suffering of that individual and economic loss to the farmer. Slaughtering or killing the PI animal will stop further virus transmission (at least from this animal). Calculating the time period when the animal was in the first trimester of foetal life will give an indication of where to trace the origin of infection.

Purpose	Target condition	Case definition	Test-result	Action/ decision
Improve welfare and profitability	Animals born immune tolerant and thus PI	Animals in which BVDV has been detected in two samples obtained at least 3 weeks apart	Detection of virus, antigen or RNA in two samples at least 3 weeks apart (blood ear notch or other)	Slaughter of the PI animal
Reduce transmission				Removing animal from the herd
Trace origin of infection				Calculate time of infection

Most BVDV infections of immuno-competent animals result in production of antibodies that are long-lasting and in most cases even lifelong. Therefore, in herds with endemic infection, many animals will be antibody positive. For these animals, there is no specific indication as to when infection occurred, only that they were infected earlier in life. Therefore, the value of such information for each individual cow is often limited. However, if the information on presence of antibodies from several cows, or maybe even all cows in the herd, is aggregated to establish an age-specific antibody profile at herd level, then valuable information on herd infection status can be given. The age distribution of antibody carriers in a herd known to be without PI animals is shown here (Reprinted from Research in Veterinary Science, 53, Houe, Serological analysis of a small herd sample to predict presence or absence of animals persistently infected with bovine virus diarrhoea virus (BVDV) in dairy herds, 320-323, Copyright (1992), with permission from Elsevier).

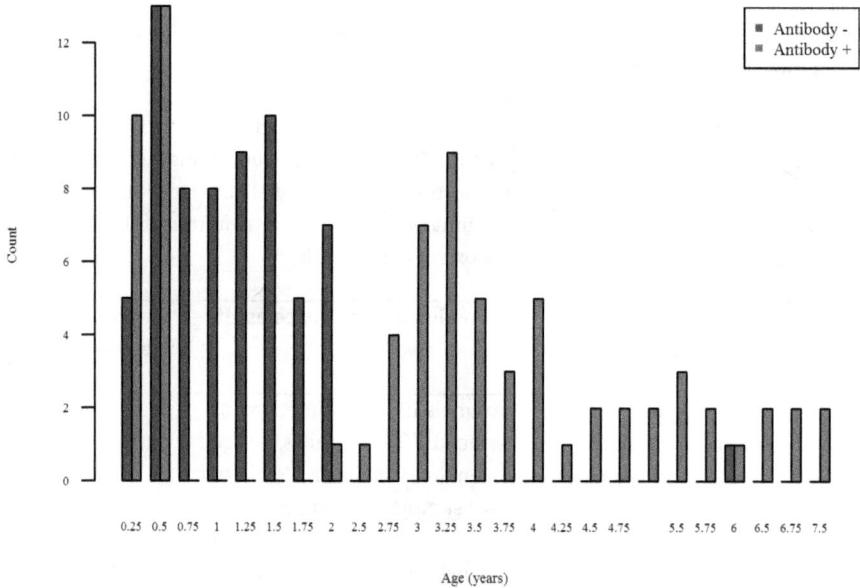

The obvious explanation for this distribution is that until approximately 3 years prior to the screening, the presence of one or more PI animals substantially increased the infection pressure, resulting in a transient infection in many animals within the herd. Old antibody-positive cows are gradually replaced by young antibody-negative animals born after removal of the PI animals. Note that many of the calves younger than 6 months are antibody-positive due to consumption of maternal antibodies via colostrum.

Thus, the pattern of antibodies according to age can serve to monitor the infection status at the herd level. Testing a cohort of ten young stock (YS) for antibodies actually

54

revealed a high Se (0.93) and Sp (1.00) for detection of herds with PI animals (Houe, 1994; Houe 1999). The target condition was whether any PI animals were present in the herd. The case definition (used in these studies) was detection of a BVDV-ELISA-positive animal among ten YS in the herd. The difference between the target condition and case definition here is that a negative case could still have non-viraemic PI animals due to colostrum. The test-result would be testing of ten YS (older than 6 months) for presence of antibodies. The action could be to classify the herd as infectious, which in a control programme would mean that positive herds would undergo follow up of individual animals, whereas negative herds could go on for continued monitoring.

Purpose	Target condition	Case definition	Test-result	Action/ decision
Monitoring herd infection status	PI animals in the herd	Detection of PI animals by whole-herd testing using ELISA	Testing ten YS (older than 6 months) for presence of antibodies	Classify herds with legislative consequences

References

Christensen J, Gardner IA, 2000. Herd-level interpretation of test results for epidemiologic studies of animal diseases. Preventive Veterinary Medicine 45:83-106.

Cornish TE, van Olphen AL, Cavender JL, Edwards JM, Jaeger PT, Vieyra LL, Woodard LF, Miller DR, O'Toole D, 2005. Comparison of ear notch immunohistochemistry, ear notch antigen-capture ELISA, and buffy coat virus isolation for detection of calves persistently infected with bovine viral diarrhea virus. Journal of Veterinary Diagnostic Investigation 17:110-117.

Houe H, 1994. Bovine virus diarrhoea virus: detection of Danish dairy herds with persistently infected animals by means of a screening test of ten young stock. Preventive Veterinary Medicine 19: 241-248.

Houe H, 1999. Epidemiological features and economical importance of bovine virus diarrhoea virus (BVDV) infections. Veterinary Microbiology 64:89-107.

Mahmmod Y, Mweu M, Nielsen SS, Katholm J, Klaas I, 2013. Effect of carryover and presampling procedures on the results of real-time PCR used for diagnosis of bovine intramammary infections with *Streptococcus agalactiae* at routine milk recordings. Preventive Veterinary Medicine 113: 512-521.

Nielsen SS, 2007. Danish control programme for bovine paratuberculosis. Cattle Practice 15: 161–168.

Nielsen SS, Houe H, Ersbøll AK, Toft N, 2004. Evaluation diagnostic tests. In: Houe H, Ersbøll AK, Toft N (Eds): Introduction to Veterinary Epidemiology. Biofolia, Frederiksberg C, Denmark.

Nielsen SS, Toft N, Gardner IA, 2011. Structured approach to design of diagnostic test evaluation studies for chronic progressive infections in animals. Veterinary Microbiology 150:115–125.

Nielsen SS, Toft N, Okura H, 2013. Dynamics of specific anti-*Mycobacterium avium* subsp. *paratuberculosis* antibody response through age. PLoS One. 8:e63009.

Nielsen TD, Nielsen LR, Toft N, 2011. Bayesian estimation of true between-herd and within-herd prevalence of *Salmonella* in Danish veal calves. Preventive Veterinary Medicine 100:155–162.

OIE, 2003. Validation and certification of diagnostic tests. OIE World Organisation for Animal Health, Paris, France. http://www.oie.int/our-scientific-expertise/registration-of-diagnostic-kits/background-information/ (accessed 24 September 2014).

OIE, 2013. OIE WAHID database on Animal Health Information. Available at: http://www.oie.int/wahis_2/public/wahid.php/Diseaseinformation/statuslist (accessed 17 May 2013).

Sergeant ES, Nielsen SS, Toft N, 2008. Evaluation of test-strategies for estimating probability of low prevalence of paratuberculosis in Danish dairy herds. Preventive Veterinary Medicine 85:92-106.

Warnick LD, Nielsen LR, Nielsen J, Greiner M, 2006. Simulation model estimates of test accuracy and predictive values for the Danish *Salmonella* surveillance program in dairy herds. Preventive Veterinary Medicine 77:284-303.

Whitlock RH, Rosenberger AE, Sweeney RW, Spencer PA, 1996. Distribution of *M. paratuberculosis* in tissues of cattle from herds infected with Johne's disease. In: Chiodini RJ, Hines II ME, Collins MT (Eds.), Proceedings of the Fifth International Colloquium on Paratuberculosis, 29 September – 04 October 1996, Madison, WI, USA, pp. 168–174.

Wilks C, 2001. Gold standards and fool's gold. Australian Veterinary Journal 79, 115.

6

The pilot project

6.1. Introduction

Control or eradication programmes are often preceded by a pilot project. In general, the main goal of a pilot project is, 'to assess feasibility so as to avoid potentially disastrous consequences of embarking on a large study' (Thabane et al., 2010). The feasibility can include: evaluation of the test-strategy; assessment to determine whether the instigated biosecurity measures will in fact prevent introduction or transmission of the pathogen; study of farmers' willingness to comply with the management of the infection; evaluation of logistics in handling infected animals; and identification of the need for communication of guidelines.

This chapter aims to demonstrate how existing scientific knowledge must be put into the context of practical experiences. Such practical experiences can be obtained from local veterinary practitioners who have tried to eradicate the infection in individual herds, or they can be more systematically obtained in larger, formal pilot projects. This chapter provides some examples of pilot projects, and outlines the associated requirements and principles.

6.2. The need for pilot projects

For most infections, a considerable number of pathogen sources and possible transmission routes are described in the literature. For BVDV infections, potential hosts include cattle, small ruminants, pigs and several species of wildlife. The documented modes of transmission of BVDV include direct contact as well as indirect contact (e.g. via needles, nose tongs, rectal gloves, live or contaminated vaccines and blood-feeding flies). When the first eradication plans were considered in Denmark, the large number of possible host species and transmission routes was of serious concern. This raised doubt as to whether it would, in practice, be possible or economically realistic to break all transmission routes (e.g. it is not possible to control all blood-feeding flies). However, for many transmission routes the practical importance was unknown, as these were only documented experimentally. Instead of initiating an eradication programme for an entire country or a large region, it can therefore be relevant to trial it in a limited geographical area, where only the most important biosecurity measures are included, in order to assess feasibility in practice. For BVDV, it was demonstrated in one of the 'island projects' that an elaborate test-strategy, including identification and slaughter of PI animals together with instigation of some specific biosecurity measures, was sufficient to stop the spread of BVDV (see later in this chapter).

6.3. Requirements for carrying out a pilot project

As with other studies, the pilot project should have a clearly defined objective. Usually, pilot projects do not aim to establish statistical significance, but instead aim to assess feasibility of project methodology, as previously mentioned. This means, for example, that important objectives are to demonstrate that the test-strategy is adequate to identify infectious animals, and that biosecurity measures are sufficient to prevent reinfection of cleared herds – or at least ensure that the number of reinfections is below a certain limit. It is important that the inclusion and exclusion criteria in the pilot project ensure the study population is similar to the target population (i.e. the population from which the disease should subsequently be eradicated if the pilot project in the study population is successful). Furthermore, the data collection method, as well as methodologies for interventions should be clearly defined and, if possible, implemented in the same way as intended within in a large population. Lastly, good scientific practice for data management (including checking data for errors) must be followed.

Concerning data analysis, it is of course preferable for a statistical evaluation to be included, e.g. to determine the probability that herds will stay free of infection for a year or more, and to include control herds. However, it may be unreasonable to expect a group of farmers not to make any changes in their infected herds for the duration of the pilot project if they hear about suggestions proposed to other farmers in the same period. Consequently, such studies often do not include an appropriate control group, but mainly include demonstration farms (example provided for *S.* Dublin in Nielsen and Nielsen, 2012).

The outcome of the pilot project is to decide whether it is feasible to initiate the project at all, and whether a large-scale project should be cancelled or continued with some modifications. It is important to bear in mind that a successful pilot project does not guarantee that a large-scale study will also be a success, but it can certainly increase the likelihood.

6.4. Examples of pilot projects with emphasis on the pilot projects related to the Danish BVDV control and eradication programme

A summary of the important facts regarding BVDV infection before the pilot project were:

- Cattle are by far the most important hosts of the infection.
- Cattle can be either transiently or persistently infected.
- Transiently infected animals show a strong and usually lifelong antibody response.
- PI animals are the main transmitters of BVDV.
- Transiently infected animals can also transmit the infection, but their role is less clear.
- Indirect transmission by humans or instruments is possible, but the importance is less clear and definite proof is difficult to establish.
- Diagnostic tests on individual animals have high Se and Sp; both for detecting animals with previous transient infection, and for detecting PI animals.
- The production losses due to BVDV infections are considerable.

In Denmark, it was also shown that the infection was widespread with practically all herds having antibody carriers and approximately half of the herds hosting PI animals (Houe and Meyling, 1991). This widespread occurrence was an important argument that a national control and eradication programme should, 'await results from preliminary control studies demonstrating their feasibility' (Bitsch and Rønsholt, 1995). Therefore, in 1992 the Danish island of Samsø was selected for a pilot project (Bitsch et al., 1994; Bitsch and Rønsholt, 1995). At the time, there were 36 dairy herds and 77 non-dairy herds on the island. Farmers were all invited to meetings, where they were informed about the project, and information on infection prophylaxis was provided. After the farmers had volunteered to participate, all animals older than 3 months were tested for the virus and antibodies, and PI animals were slaughtered before the pasture season. Animals younger than 3 months at the time of initial screening were dealt with in the following period. All young animals from confirmed problem herds were tested, whereas in other herds only spot samples of animals were tested. At these follow-up investigations, additional PI animals were found in three herds. These findings were not surprising, because in one herd PI calves had previously been identified, and in the two other herds, the PI animals had either been foetuses or younger than 3 months at the initial screening. As there was no further spread of BVDV, it was concluded that transmission had ceased after removal of PI animals and thereafter a general control and eradication programme seemed feasible.

Following this, an additional desire to reduce the programme cost was expressed. In particular, there was an inclination to avoid whole-herd testing of all herds. Some studies had indicated that testing a few young stock (YS) for antibodies was sufficient to predict presence or absence of PI animals. Moreover, it was shown that levels of antibodies in bulk milk were much higher in herds with PI animals than in herds without PI animals (Houe, 1993; Houe, 1994). Therefore, additional pilot projects were performed, including all dairy herds on the islands of Bornholm (n=148) and Mors (n=221), to determine the feasibility of using antibody measurements in bulk tank milk (BTM) samples for classification of herds into either having or not having PI animals (Bitsch et al., 1994; Bitsch and Rønsholt, 1995). The island of Mors was chosen to be representative of Denmark generally, whereas the other island (Bornholm) was expected to have low occurrence (Bitsch et al., 1994). These projects showed that the BTM antibody test had high Se for identification of herds with PI animals (Bitsch et al., 1994; Houe 1999).

The main conclusions from the described pilot projects were:

- Biosecurity measures must focus on avoiding direct contact with PI animals (testing of animals before admission to herds).
- Purchased animals should be isolated for 3 weeks, and newly acquired pregnant animals should be isolated and offspring tested.

- Animals should not be pastured if there is a possibility that PI animals are present in neighbouring fields.
- Common pastures, animal exhibitions and livestock markets should be free of PI animals.
- The costs of the programme can be reduced by combining BTM testing with follow-up testing of a spot sample of a few individual animals to clarify infection status of the herd, followed by testing of individual animals only in those herds still suspected of having PI animals.
- Communication to obtain farmer compliance to guidelines is crucial.

Thus, the pilot projects helped to ascertain that the control programme, including a test-strategy using a limited number of samples, was feasible. Furthermore, it seemed that most emphasis should be on avoiding contact with PI animals.

It can be debated whether an island is an appropriate selection for a pilot project of a programme intended for an entire country. It is clearly recommended that the population included in a pilot project should be representative of the target population. There may be reason to believe that this is not the case for an animal population on an island. Although not explicitly stated in the pilot project, there are several practical advantages of choosing an island. For example: it is much easier to keep control of animal movements to the area; it is very easy to define who should participate; and it may be easier to gain local political support among the farming organisations. However, when generalising from such a pilot project, it is very important that these special circumstances are acknowledged in the main project, for example by strict demands for certificates of freedom from disease when moving animals between herds.

For comparison, a more recent pilot project was established in Somerset, United Kingdom, which is one of the most cattle-dense areas in the UK (Booth and Brownlie, 2012). The pilot project identified important reasons for failure to control and eradicate BVDV, including lack of farmer participation, lack of compliance with biosecurity and testing protocols, and participating farmers leaving the project (Barrett, 2012; Booth and Brownlie, 2012). Thus, it was apparent that a number of sociological problems should be addressed before a larger project was launched.

References

Barrett D, 2012. BVD eradication: lessons from a pilot scheme. Veterinary Record 170: 71-72.

Bitsch V, Houe H, Rønsholt L, Madsen KF, Valbak J, Roug NH, Eckhardt CH, 1994. På vej mod kontrol af BVD. Dansk Veterinærtidsskrift 77: 445-450 (in Danish with English summary).

Bitsch V, Rønsholt, L, 1995. Control of bovine viral diarrhea virus infection without vaccines. Veterinary Clinics of North America. Food Animal Practice 11:627-640.

Booth RE, Brownlie J, 2012. Establishing a pilot bovine viral diarrhea virus eradication scheme in Somerset. Veterinary Record 170: 73-79.

Houe H, Meyling A, 1991. Prevalence of bovine virus diarrhoea (BVD) in 19 Danish dairy herds and estimation of incidence of infection in early pregnancy. Preventive Veterinary Medicine 11: 9-16.

Houe H, 1992. Serological analysis of a small herd sample to predict presence or absence of animals persistently infected with bovine virus diarrhoea virus (BVDV) in dairy herds. Research in Veterinary Science 53: 320-323.

Houe H, 1994. Bovine virus diarrhoea virus: Detection of Danish dairy herds with persistently infected animals by means of a screening test of ten young stock. Preventive Veterinary Medicine 19: 241-248.

Houe H, 1999. Epidemiological features and economical importance of bovine virus diarrhoea virus (BVDV). Veterinary Microbiology 64: 89-107.

Nielsen LR, Nielsen SS, 2012. A structured approach to control of *Salmonella* Dublin in 10 Danish dairy herds based on risk scoring and test-and-manage procedures. Food Research International 45: 1158-1165.

Thabane L, Ma J, Chu R, Cheng J, Ismaila A, Rios LP, Robson R, Thabane M, Giangregorio L, Goldsmith CH, 2010. A tutorial on pilot studies: the what, why and how. BMC Medical Research Methodology 10: 1.

7

Resources

7.1. Introduction

On a global scale, there are obviously large differences in availability
and prioritisation of resources, and hence also differences in whether
individual farmers, agricultural sectors and governments can and will
allocate resources for an eradication programme. However, in many
developed countries, there would be sufficient resources to back up a
decision to eradicate a disease from the country as long as all the
previously mentioned preconditions are in place.

Still, there are important differences that impact whether a decision on
national eradication of an infection will be made. In some countries,
farmers have a long tradition of being organised in one or a few
common and strong unions. This enables them to take decisions upon
eradication programmes and to implement effective initiatives to
approach the goal. The government may not need to get involved until
the late or final stages of the programmes. In other countries, individual
farmers are much more independent, or there may be many different
smaller organisations with conflicting interests. However, when
eradicating infectious diseases, it is important that decisions are made
at higher level than the individual herds. This is because infected herds
are not only a risk to themselves, but also to other herds in their
geographical area and those coming into contact with animals or
contaminated fomites from them. Furthermore, non-infected herds will
often become more susceptible as prevalence is reduced, and severe
outbreaks may occur in these herds upon new introduction of the
infectious agent. Therefore, it is often necessary that all farmers in the
same region go for the same decision of either eradicating the infection,
or living with the endemic occurrence while trying to reduce the
economic and health impact of the disease. History has shown that even
in countries with strong farmer organisations, it is necessary that the

government supports the eradication programme with appropriate legislation to ensure that all farmers comply with the risk mitigating rules of the programme.

This chapter aims to address the question 'How can eradication programmes be organised once the decision to eradicate has been made?' This covers administrative unit(s), logistics and data flow, knowledge dissemination, legislation and financial engagements supporting the common goal of eradication.

7.2. Administrative unit

The success of an eradication programme strongly relies on one or more capable administrative units, which not only possesses the required manpower, with knowledge about the pathogenesis and dynamics of the disease, but also has a thorough understanding of how to interpret laboratory test-results. Furthermore, the unit should have full access to data collected in the programme and be able to analyse surveillance data to take appropriate and timely actions when needed. It is important that the administrative unit of the programme is able to fulfil the tasks over an extended period of time (i.e. several years or even decades) and that farmers generally have a sufficient level of trust in the administration. Of course the administrators also have to know the relevant legislation in detail. Typically administrators of national eradication programmes have also been involved in the formulation and establishment of the programme including the regulation. The administrative unit can be organisationally located in an independent public or private animal health institution, a private farmer organisation, a national veterinary authority or a national veterinary laboratory. It is important that farmers, their local advisors and laboratories involved in the programme know how to contact the administrative unit, and that it is easy to reach. The administrative unit can take different sizes and the amounts of support it will need to offer to individual farmers vary. In some programmes or during some phases of the programme, the administrative unit handles the actual herd classification system and restrictions implied by classifications including paperwork, database management and associated communication, but the needed local advisory functions are handled by local herd health advisors. In other cases or during other phases of the programme, the administrative unit may be very involved in providing detailed advisory service and makes visits to infected farms in need of specialised counselling. Depending on how many farms are infected each year, this can have a huge effect on the resources needed for administration. It also varies between countries how much of the expenses for administration and advisory functions are covered by public or common private farmer funds, and how much has to be paid by the individual farmers.

In Denmark, the administration of the national surveillance, control and eradication programmes for BVDV, *S.* Dublin and paratuberculosis are placed centrally at the Knowledge Centre for Agriculture, which belongs under one large agricultural organisation, the Danish Agriculture & Food Council. There, a group of specialised veterinarians and technical assistants work in close collaboration with the Danish Veterinary and Food Administration, and the relevant laboratories and research institutions to continuously follow and respond to issues arising during the eradication phases. The advisory functions regarding elimination of infections in the individual farms are mainly the responsibility of the local veterinarians, and to some extent the regional cattle-farming advisory services. However, individual farmers or local advisors may ask for either publicly or self-funded assistance from the central administrative unit when faced with persistent infections or new, severe outbreaks of infections. In other countries, these responsibilities and functions are taken care of by independent private institutions with veterinary laboratory facilities and advisory services for the farmers.

7.3. Logistics and flow of data

Large-scale programmes require considerations on large-scale management of diagnostic data, diagnostic information, communication of test-results, provision of other information and education to train the users in the mindset behind the programme. These may be managed by the administrative unit, but can also be outsourced and managed separately. Generally, common systems, definitions, terminology, tests etc. are required to ensure that all stakeholders are in agreement about all of the essential approaches used in the control and eradication programme. A common system could for instance be the practice of using milk samples already collected for quality assurance purposes for systematic animal level or herd level testing and classification used together with a set of recommendations about how to interpret the test-results and the resulting animal or herd classifications (e.g. 'red, yellow and green cow classifications' upon testing of milk samples with paratuberculosis ELISA).

<u>Laboratory facilities</u>

Most programmes include diagnostic information and consequently also rely on the capabilities of diagnostic laboratories. For example, a programme cannot be dependent on large-scale pathological investigations, if there are no facilities to carry out post-mortem examinations, and no staff trained to do it. Another example: bacteriological culture of faecal samples to detect MAP may require assessment of say four 10ml tubes taking up space equivalent of about 10cm^2. A sample should be cultured about 3 months in a room a temperature of 37°C to ensure MAP growth, so four batches can be done in a year. Therefore, samples from 100,000 cows would require about 25,000 x 10cm^2 = 2,500m^2 of incubator shelf space per year, if each cow was sampled once. In Denmark, there are two or three laboratories that can do the analyses, but none of them have incubator capacity of that magnitude. Of course, it is possible to create such space. The point is that it needs to be thought of in the planning process.

Blood samples are easy to draw from individuals. Large-scale sampling will require a lot of manpower, and might require education of technicians to do so. However, not all organisations will approve of technicians drawing blood, e.g. the Danish Veterinary Association or animal protection groups might oppose to blood being drawn from livestock without 'proper training', which again might be defined as having a veterinary degree. This on the other hand may increase the expenses in the programme. Therefore, if such sampling should be carried out, stakeholders should be contacted to sense their views on the possibilities and different scenarios.

In many countries, milk recording is carried out in a proportion of the national cattle population on a regular basis. The resulting milk samples might be used, if they are already in the pipeline of the laboratories, e.g. for monitoring of production or herd health. Perhaps transfer from one laboratory to another is necessary, but it is easier with two locations than with hundreds. Therefore, milk samples might offer a possibility as a diagnostic specimen, if they have already been collected. However, use of milk recording samples will exclude those outside the milk recording scheme and non-dairy herds which need to be considered as well. Another challenge is the possible cross-contamination of samples, which may be a bigger problem in relation to agent detecting tests such as PCR-based tests than to indirect tests such as antibody ELISAs.

Therefore, logistics of sampling and testing are pivotal to consider in the course of programme planning. Once the test materials are in the laboratories, it is beneficial that all laboratories use the same test. The individual laboratory might have their view on what 'the best test' is, and consequently do not use the same as others. Programme managers could make it a requirement that all use the same test – for comparative purposes and in order to do statistics across all enrolled herds and animals. This may be more important than a few per cent point gains in diagnostic sensitivity (Se).

Data flow and ownership

The diagnostic data resulting from the programme should be used by farmers and herd health advisors for daily management and decisions (Fig. 7.1). Processed and interpreted laboratory reports for such decisions should inform the same type of decisions in all types of herds, irrespective of the origin of the test-results. Report standardisation can therefore also be a benefit. One way of assuring that is to use a central database with central reporting system serving all end users, see an example of a standardised report from the Danish paratuberculosis control programme in Fig. 7.2.

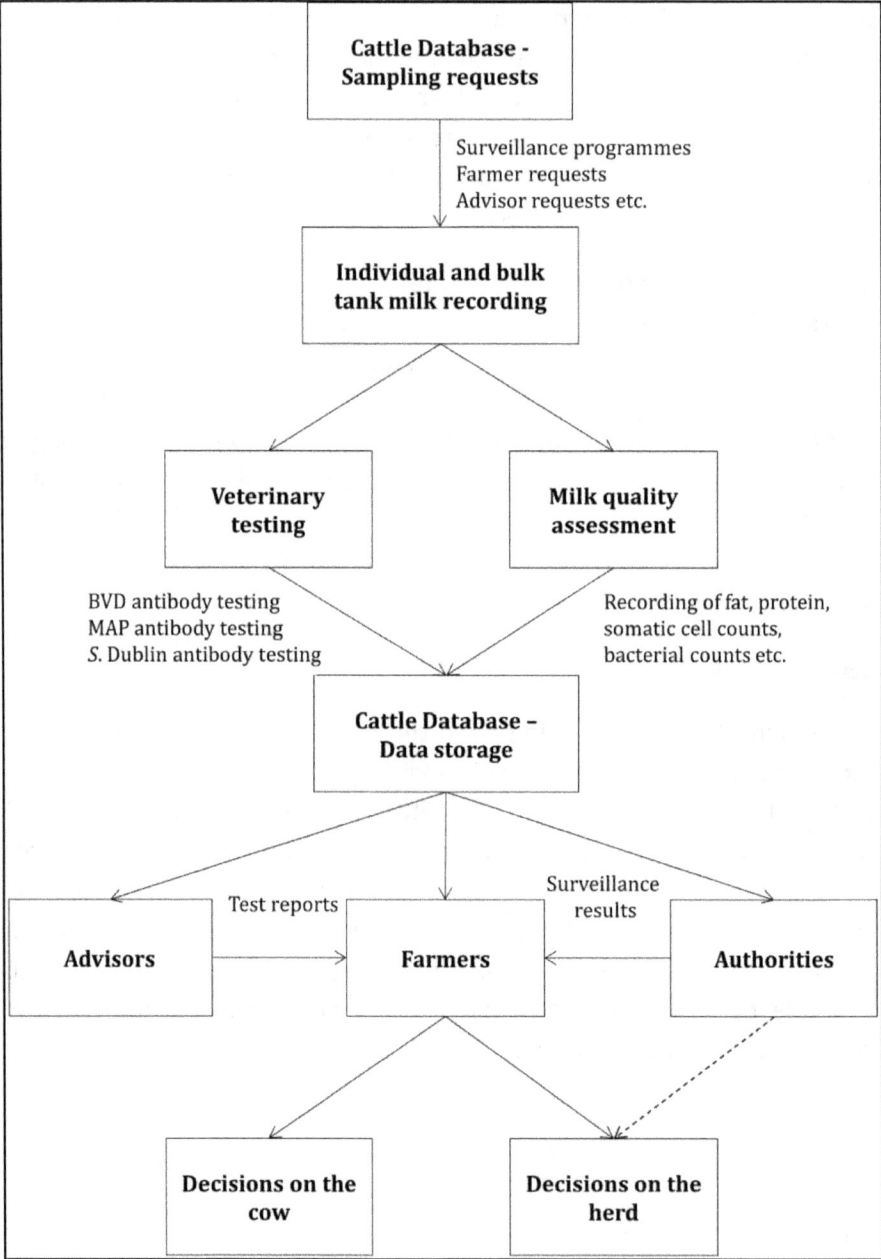

Figure 7.1. From data to decision: Chart on selected data flow in the Danish Cattle Database.

The diagnostic data should also be used to inform progress (or lack of same) in the programme, e.g. for prevalence estimates. This is only feasible if the data are collected at national or regional level. If such data are collected, the data flow should be considered. Furthermore, the ownership of the data should be resolved, and it should be agreed for which purposes the data can be used by different stakeholders such as farmers, herd health advisors, researchers and authorities.

ParaTB Management list for Herd Y by 04 June 2014. Only valid until 04 October 2014.

High-risk cows: High level of hygiene around calving; No use of milk and colostrum

Animal ID	ELISA 1 06.04.14	Previous 26.02.14	Parity	Expected calving	Production loss	Antibody group
1052	0.2	.	7		Possible	3
1107	0.0	0.1	4		Possible	3
1188	0.2	0.3	4		Possible	3
1219	1.1	1.6	4		Very likely	5
1310	0.0	0.1	3		Possible	3
1345	0.6	0.1	2	05.08.14	Likely	4
1408	0.0	0.3	1		Possible	3
1414	2.2	2.7	2		Very likely	5
1441	2.6	3.5	1	13.10.14	Very likely	5

Low-risk cows: Colostrum and milk can be used for feeding of heifer-calves

Animal ID	ELISA 1 06.04.14	Previous 26.02.14	Parity	Expected calving	Production loss	Antibody group
1024	0.0	0.2	6		Not likely	1
1078	0.0	0.0	5	26.10.14	Not likely	1
1080	0.0	.	6		Not likely	1
1116	0.0	0.1	5		Not likely	1
1145	0.0	0.0	5		Not likely	1

Figure 7.2. Standardised report used in the Danish paratuberculosis control programme for management and culling of cows tested in the programme (e.g. 'red cows' are recommended for culling immediately, 'yellow cows' are recommended to be managed as potential shedders of MAP in milk and faeces).

In Denmark, most data ends up in the Danish Cattle Database (managed by the Knowledge Centre for Agriculture), which is linked up to the Danish Central Husbandry Register containing information on demographics of all livestock. The general rule is that data are owned by the individual farmer, and cannot be used by anybody without the farmer's consent, except for summary statistics and the like in anonymised form and for some specified research purposes. This ensures that the data can be used for motivation of farmers as a whole in a programme, but also that the data can be used for further development of a programme. This promotes a continuous awareness.

Data actually follows the individual cow. Consequently, if a cow has a previous diagnosis, this information follows the cow and is available to a new owner as well to a new herd health advisor. This makes it difficult to hide former 'defects' that might be deemed to reduce the value of the trade good (the traded cow). This makes cheating more difficult, and if cheating is difficult and likely to be discovered, then appropriate behaviour may be promoted and exerted.

7.4. Knowledge dissemination and continuing education

The educational level among all involved parties is rarely sufficiently high or uniform to carry out a programme, prior to the programme being initiated. A high level should ensure that farmers and herd health advisors have sufficient knowledge of how to control the spread of the infection. A uniform level should ensure that information can be distributed in a terminology similar to everybody, including all stakeholders (see Chapter 9).

The knowledge to be disseminated and best practice advised should also be agreed upon. There might be several 'best practices', but mixing them may not always be desirable. Therefore, a single strategy for the entire programme can be adopted as an official strategy, even though for some farmers an alternative strategy may appear more beneficial. This ensures that alternatives are made on the responsibility of the individual. One example is that low antibody measurements of all blood samples from ten randomly selected calves between 3-6 months old form a general recommended criterion to evaluate the effect of hygiene and management practices for breaking the most important part of the transmission cycle of *S.* Dublin in cattle herds. However, there may be some herds with little spread among young calves that would benefit from an alternative focus and testing strategy such as testing of heifers close to calving or adult cows to detect suspected persistently infected carriers for culling. Conversely, if this was recommended to all herds, it would be an expensive and not very effective solution seen from the perspective of the entire programme. This challenges the local advisors, who have to be able to keep the overall aim of the programme in sight, while still being able to provide effective, herd-specific advice. A good herd health advisor should be able to understand and appreciate the benefit of both general recommendations, and specific needs and situations in some herds, and his/her advisory services should consequently be herd-specific.

Knowledge upgrade for farmers and herd health advisors can be done via:

- Courses for those requiring courses;
- Information material for those believing they can do self-study;
- Participatory methods such as experience groups.

Being prescriptive about having to take specific courses may be used as an approach, but can also backfire. For example, course participants may lose interest in the vital parts and start focusing on less essential elements, merely to prove to course leaders or programme administrators that there are other approaches that could be used to control the infection. Furthermore, people are different and some learn better via self-study or learning-by-doing, if appropriate materials and information are made available. Others may learn better at structured courses. In recent years, participatory methods for knowledge dissemination, stimulated self-learning and implementation of control strategies have become popular, e.g. stable schools for farmers (Anon., 2008; Shiferaw et al., 2010; Vaarst et al., 2007). Combining these approaches should therefore increase the general knowledge level.

7.5. Legislation

Voluntary programmes and mandatory programmes may have different needs for guidelines and use of legislation in different phases. There will always be farmers lacking the interest or need to comply with the recommendations. If their herds are or become infected, they will be a major threat to surrounding herds that are susceptible. However, the government has an interest in waiting as long as possible before intervening, not least due to the fact that demands in legislation may be costly for the government in manpower resources and payments for testing and culling of animals. Also, if follow-up investigations (see Chapter 10) show that there are weaknesses in biosecurity or test-strategies, it may be necessary to strengthen legislation over time. A very important part of both the general and disease-specific legislation is the placement of responsibility in case an infected animal is traded. If for example, farmers can be held responsible for infecting another herd by selling an infected animal, it will certainly impact compliance with all the rules of the programme.

7.6. Finances

It should be obvious from the above sections that financial coverage of expenses is an issue that needs to be addressed early on and continuously during a national eradication programme. Several stakeholders may have to cover the expenses of different parts of the programme. The stakeholders differ to some extent depending on the disease in question. Therefore, the financial coverage may differ between programmes. For instance, if an infection is zoonotic the government may be more willing to cover some of the financial needs than if the disease solely affects animal health and production. At a national level, the expenses for the programme activities should be seen in relation to the losses caused by the disease, but it should also be realised that it may not be the same stakeholders that will pay for the programme activities as those who will benefit from the disease being eradicated from the country. To give an idea about which elements to consider when budgeting for eradication programmes, an example of financial elements are summarised below for the Danish *S.* Dublin programme and weighted against other economic considerations of relevance for *S.* Dublin in the cattle sector.

Table 7.1. This summarises costs revealed in a report to the Danish Minister for Food, Agriculture and Fisheries written by a scientific and technical advisory group for the *S.* Dublin programme development in 2009 (Anon, 2009). The reported total costs for the eradication programme activities during the 6-year period 2009-2014 were almost EUR 14 million (equivalent to EUR 2.3 million per year).

Activity	Period	Financed by	Amount in EUR per year
Surveillance (sampling, laboratory analyses and IT/database maintenance and programme administration)	2010-2014	Cattle and Milk Levy Funds (before 2010 85% of the expenses were covered by so-called CO_2 funds, a tax that was collected from farmers and returned by the government to the farming industry for beneficial projects)	~0.4 million
Eradication/field activities (Pilot project, stable schools, IT-development, advisory group work)		Cattle and Milk Levy Funds	~1 million
Projects about slaughter hygiene		34% Cattle Levy Fund 66% foreign abattoirs + other funding sources	>160,000
Danish Veterinary and Food Administration (administration of legislation)	2010-2014	Government funding	~22,250
National Veterinary and Food Institutes (scientific and laboratory advice / reference lab work)	2010-2014	Government funding	~22,250
Case by case surveillance of meat	2009-2010	Government funding	~100,000
Research projects concerning development of surveillance methods, food safety evaluation, evaluation of effects of eradication at herd level, development of new diagnostic methods, evaluation of bacterial contamination at abattoirs	2009-2011	About 50% government funding and about 50% the Cattle and Milk Levy Funds	~ 800,000
Estimated costs of control activities in infected herds (based on an estimated 600 herds having to eradicate the infection and average expenses for testing, culling, new/reconstructions of barns, investments, advisory services)	2009-2014	Farmers' own expenses	1.3 million

Actual cost-benefit or cost-effectiveness estimations have not been carried out for each of the activities. Therefore, they must be evaluated in the light of the overall reduction in prevalence of *S*. Dublin test-positive Danish dairy herds from 14% in January 2009 to 8% in January 2014. They could also be seen as part of a long-term investment in securing safe food that is free from *S*. Dublin bacteria.

Costs related to hospitalisation and lost lives to *S*. Dublin infections in humans were not considered here and they are largely unknown. Furthermore, rough estimates of the economic losses caused by acute and endemic *S*. Dublin infections in the Danish dairy herds at the national prevalence level in 2012 amounted to more than DKK 52 million (EUR 7 million) per year based on economic losses estimated at herd level by Nielsen et al. (2013). However, these estimates are of interest to farmers and farmer organisations more than consumers. As also covered in Chapters 3 and 9, these aspects once again emphasise the different stakeholders, their roles, potential benefits and the fact that not all benefits can be quantified, but resources to cover all costs are still required.

References

Anonymous, 2008. Evaluering af pilotprojekt *Salmonella* Syd- og Sønderjylland. *In*: Nielsen LR (Ed.), Mejeriforeningen, Afdeling for Veterinære forhold og Råvarekvalitet, Frederiks Alle 22, 8000 Århus C, pp. 1-91.

Anonymous, 2009. Handlingsplan for *Salmonella* Dublin i kvæg. The Danish Veterinary and Food Administration, Mørkhøj, Denmark. www.fvst.dk, (accessed 24 September 2014).

Nielsen TD, Kudahl AB, Østergaard S, Nielsen LR, 2013. Gross margin losses due to *Salmonella* Dublin infection in Danish dairy cattle herds estimated by simulation modelling. Preventive Veterinary Medicine 111: 51-62.

Shiferaw TJ, Moses K, Manyahilishal KE, 2010. Participatory appraisal of foot and mouth disease in the Afar pastoral area, northeast Ethiopia: implications for understanding disease ecology and control strategy. Tropical Animal Health and Production 42: 193-201.

Vaarst M, Nissen TB, Østergaard S, Klaas IC, Bennedsgaard TW, Christensen J, 2007. Danish stable schools for experiential common learning in groups of organic dairy farmers. Journal of Dairy Science 90: 2543-2554.

8

Deciding upon the initiation of a systematic control and eradication programme

8.1. Introduction

This chapter combines all the information on motivation, biosecurity, test-strategies, resources, legislation etc. from previous chapters. It sets up a framework to envisage all the relevant information needed for a decision on eradication. In the case of a particular disease, it is rarely possible to fulfil all the requirements outlined. Therefore, the relevant knowledge pertaining to the eradication of each individual disease should be considered in terms of its strengths and weaknesses. The idea is that a 'profile' for the infection can be established. This means that although any evaluation of a disease should address all elements mentioned in this book, the final basis for the decision will differ from one disease to another. As an example, for BVDV, the eradication programme can place emphasis on test-strategies and animal movement since there is limited survival of the pathogen in the environment, and highly accurate tests exist. Survival of the pathogen in the environment is considerably higher for *S.* Dublin and MAP, and as a result there is a greater need to include a number of biosecurity management procedures associated with the environment and indirect transmission. These examples illustrate some overall differences, but when systematically reviewing all the 'elements needed for control and eradication', a specific profile for each disease can be established.

The compiled biological knowledge needs to be put into a socioeconomic context. A disease with moderate financial impact may be eligible for eradication if it is technically straightforward to do. Conversely, a disease with difficult technical challenges (e.g. in breaking transmission) may be eligible for eradication if there are significant associated economic losses, or if the infection is zoonotic.

The chapter is structured to address the following questions:

WHY is it important or relevant to control this infection?

WHAT should be done to control and eradicate?

WHICH knowledge gaps still exist?

WHO should be involved and informed, and HOW should the programme be organised?

WHERE should the programme be implemented?

WHICH measures (test systems) should be used to monitor progress?

WHEN have control and eradication been achieved?

For each question, the relevant information must be extracted from literature, experts and other sources. Hereafter, the information should be checked for validity as well as feasibility for inclusion in a programme. This way, the overall principles from evidence-based medicine are followed.

8.2. WHY is it important or relevant to control this infection?

A decision maker often considers the magnitude and importance of the problem first. This question is discussed in detail in Chapter 3, where it is illustrated that a disease can be deemed important for different reasons. For example, a disease that causes moderate losses on average can be deemed important if it can occasionally have devastating effects. In addition to direct economic losses, diseases that have animal welfare or food safety implications have high relevance, due to change in consumer attitudes and consequently to product demand. Therefore, the answer to this question arises from a debate among many stakeholders. The different implications of the disease commonly affect the farmer, and hence the farmers' incentives. This is illustrated in the following flow charts:

Production losses -> Economic implication for farmers and difficult working conditions

Welfare implications -> Negative consumer attitude -> Lower market share -> Economic losses

Food safety implications -> Negative consumer attitude -> Lower market share -> Economic losses

In addition, some zoonotic diseases may lead to societal burdens due to hospitalisations and lost working capacity, if people become infected.

The flow charts illustrate that the control and eradication of diseases often are advantageous from several viewpoints and hence for several stakeholders.

8.3. WHAT should be done to control and eradicate?
The overall question must be developed further into sub-questions so that the answers can be used directly as actions in the programme. One of the most relevant questions is: How can we stop transmission of infection? Some of the central information regarding this question (outlined in Chapter 4) is compiled in Table 8.1.

In parallel with breaking the transmission routes, a purpose-specific test-strategy must be established. Table 8.2 provides a summary of the important elements outlined in Chapter 5.

Table 8.1. How can we stop transmission of the pathogen?

What do we know and what tools do we have?	What should be done (with this knowledge)?
Diagnostic tests to identify infectious hosts.	Identify infection status of possible infectious hosts and latent carriers that may become infectious.
	Depending on the speed of the programme: - Restrict animal movements from the farm (no trade, sharing pasture or animal shows). - Slaughter or 'euthanise and destroy' relevant animals.
	Quarantine or isolate animals entering the herd; or obtain test certificates.
Existence of reservoir hosts.	Avoid contact between reservoir host and primary host.
Possible indirect transmission routes.	Establish hygienic precautions for visitors and vehicles. Establish insect and rodent control, restrict access to barns for dogs, cats etc.
Survival of pathogen in the environment.	Break within-herd transmission, e.g. via improved hygiene of calving pens, separation of cows and calves, separate use of equipment in different herd sections.
	Break between-herd transmission, e.g. through extra awareness of above-mentioned indirect transmission routes including shared equipment and spread of manure.

Table 8.2. Purpose and use of a specific test-strategy.

What do we know?	What should be done (with the test information)?
Sensitivity (Se) and specificity (Sp) for different (relevant) infection stages of primary host species.	Reduce transmission from infectious animals. Remove infectious animals from the herd. If possible, create test certificates for animals to be moved.
Se and Sp for tests or combination of tests for identification of infected herds (with no prior knowledge of infection).	Classify herds in infection categories, for example: a) Non-infected b) Infection suspected c) Infected.
Se and Sp of herd tests in recently cleared herds.	Monitor recently cleared herds.
Se and Sp of herd tests in disease-free herds.	Monitor disease-free herds.

8.4. WHICH knowledge gaps still exist?

After all the technical aspects of breaking transmission and establishing a test-strategy have been outlined, it is time to identify whether there are important gaps in our existing knowledge of the infection. Therefore, it is important to evaluate whether all the activities listed in the second column of Tables 8.1 and 8.2 are sufficiently established in the scientific literature. Examples of knowledge gaps and suggestions to solve them are given in Table 8.3.

Table 8.3. Examples of knowledge gaps when undertaking the necessary activities in a control and eradication programme.

Activity	Knowledge gap	Possible solution
Avoid contact between reservoir host and primary host	The actual occurrence among e.g. deer may be unknown	Perform a screening in collaboration with hunters
Insect and rodent control	It may be known from experimental studies that transmission via flies is possible, but the practical implication is unknown	Make a pilot project without insect control
Monitor infection-free herds	It may not be known whether a bulk tank milk (BTM) test has sufficient Se to detect herds with only one infected cow	Make diagnostic test of diluted milk to establish the Se of BTM testing or compare within-herd prevalence with BTM results

8.5. WHO should be involved and informed, how should the programme be organised, and WHERE should the programme be implemented?

As research on different elements of the preconditions and criteria for control and eradication programmes often evolve over time (see Fig. 2.1), so may the organisation undergo considerable changes. In all phases of the programme, it is important to outline all the possible key players. These key players may have different levels of motivation for their engagement, and will therefore differ in their willingness to contribute time and resources to the programme.

86

The key players often include:

- Farmers
- Farmers' organisations
- Veterinary practitioners / herd health advisors and their organisations
- Veterinary laboratories
- Authorities: Veterinary and Food Administration / Government
- Research institutions

The overall engagement of the different parties will determine whether participation in the programme will be voluntary or mandatory. This may affect the effectiveness of the programme.

As outlined in Chapter 7, the different activities of a programme can be placed at governmental institutions, farmers' organisations or even outsourced to private companies. The affiliation can vary substantially depending on the traditions of different countries. An important requirement of a systematic control programme is that all decisions and activities are clearly organised and allocated between the different institutions and organisations. Which specific institution or organisation actually performs the activity may be of minor concern. Furthermore, the programme organisation may also evolve over time. Fig. 8.1 schematically shows two different examples. In Example A, there is a bottom-up pressure from farmers and local veterinarians pushing for a coordinated effort. This prompts the farmers' organisations to establish a more coordinated effort including a programme administration to handle data and provide general advice to farmers and practitioners. Over time, the government can support the initiative by creating new legislation forcing farmers to comply with at least some of the recommendations in the programme. In example B, the initiative and decisions are clearly top-down, with the government creating legislation, the veterinary authorities controlling the programme and the farmers and practitioners making the necessary interventions within the herds. Example B can represent situations with zoonotic infections or eradication programmes that are well underway or close to completion. Note that Fig. 8.1 is a very simplified diagram as there are many feedback loops in the system; and the programme organisation in example A may gradually change to the organisation structure in example B.

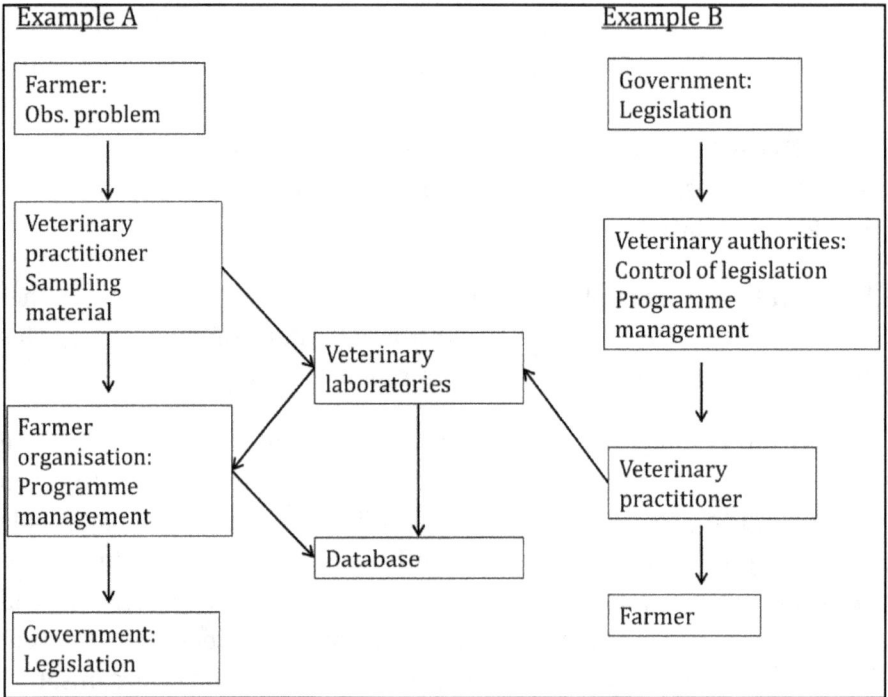

Figure 8.1. Schematic outline of two examples of programme organisation.

The Danish programmes on BVDV and paratuberculosis were initiated as bottom-up processes, where farmers required initiatives to deal with a problem specific to an individual herd (Chapter 11). The main problems in these cases were reduced animal health (e.g. abortions and diarrhoea), and loss of profitability. The *S.* Dublin programme was, on the other hand, initiated primarily to deal with a zoonotic issue. A top-down process was primarily put in place, motivated by politicians concerned with public health. None of the programmes were fully bottom-up or top-down, because in practice they were 'rolling forward and backward' until 'consensus' had been achieved. Such changes in the programme organisation will naturally affect which herds and regions are included in the programme.

8.6. WHICH measures (test systems) should be used to monitor progress?

To a large extent, progress can be monitored by compiling all the data provided by the test-strategy as outlined in Chapter 5 and Table 8.2. Graphs can then be made of each of the infection categories (non-infected, suspected and infected), or can illustrate the estimated true prevalence of infected herds as shown in Fig. 11.3.2. The incidence of new infections in herds that have already been cleared is also important in measuring progress. However, as will be explained later in Chapter 10, an eradication programme is dynamic and the testing regime may need to be modified as the programme progresses. Any change in the testing regime used for monitoring progress should be transparent. Hence, prevalence measures at different time points (e.g. one or two years apart) may not be directly comparable, and if data are not carefully interpreted both overestimation and underestimation of the progress is possible. It is an advantage if accurate estimations of Se and Sp of tests and test-strategies (both at individual animal level and at herd level) are provided repeatedly during the eradication programme.

8.7. WHEN have control and eradication been achieved?

This question can be seen as the final conclusion of the previous sections, and is also central to the decision to favour eradication over control. It is recommended that establishing a profile for the infection should be integral to making any final decision. Table 8.4 summarises some relevant characteristics for control (impact, biosecurity and test performance) of the three different diseases used as examples in this book.

Table 8.4. Disease characteristics of relevance for control (impact, transmission and test performance) for three different diseases.

Disease characteristics of relevance for control		Infection		
		BVDV	**_S._ Dublin**	**PTB**
Impact	Animal welfare	XXX	X	XX
	Farming profitability	XXX	XX	XX
	Zoonotic potential	0	XXX	X?
Biosecurity	Infection likely via live animals	XXX	XX	XX
	Spread via environment	X	XXX	XXX
Test performance	Test performance of individual animals' infection status	XXX	XX	X
	Accurate herd-level diagnosis	XXX	XX	(X)

It can be seen from Table 8.4 that the three diseases score very differently on different characteristics. Therefore, the conclusion regarding eligibility of a disease for eradication can be based on very different combinations of these characteristics. These characteristics should be considered together with the evidence or validity of the information. In this way, it is transparent in the final decision, if some shortcomings exist, and whether interested parties should be willing to take some risk. The circumstances for making the final decision can be seen as the balance of two sides of a scale – on the one side are all the advantages (financial, animal welfare, food safety) and on the other side the hesitation and concerns over its feasibility. It may also be seen as the 'weight' of influential people on 'the yes side' and on 'the no side'. Table 8.5 summarises the questions. A final decision to aim for eradication should specify a target year in which the disease 'for all practical purposes' can be considered eradicated. This approach was taken for the Danish _S._ Dublin programme in which the target point for eradication initially was specified as the 'end of 2014' (Chapter 11.3.8) and later adjusted to the 'end of 2016' (Chapter 11.3.9).

Table 8.5. Profile of a disease, addressing different 'WH'-questions

Question	Common answers, reasons, options or things to consider
WHY	Farming profitability; animal welfare; animal health; food safety
WHAT	Needs to be considered about pathogen survival; biosecurity measure feasibility; test performance and test-strategies
WHICH	Essential knowledge gaps exist related to control or eradication; occurrence in wild life; possible air borne transmission
WHO	Are the stakeholders and key players, how should they be organised, and how should programme be initiated (bottom-up; top-down)
WHERE	Local, regional, national, international efforts
WHICH	Tests and surveillance methods should be used to measure progress; modification of test regimen over time
WHEN	Is the target year for control and/or eradication

8.8. Example: Case – BVDV eradication in Denmark

In the years before the BVDV eradication programme in Denmark was established, there was intensive debate at meetings and in magazines about whether sufficient information to start an eradication programme existed. Some practitioners argued that they had successfully eradicated the infection in several of their cattle herds and therefore a national programme should be initiated (Katholm and Markman 1994). However, others argued that even though the infection could be successfully eradicated in some herds, this might not be the case in all herds. Thus, they doubted whether the initial success stories could be generalised to the whole country, as it could have just been the most collaborative farmers who participated in the first 'herd-level programmes'. Opponents to a programme also put forward a very long list of possible transmission routes – some of which were later considered to be of minor importance. An example of the debates from the newspapers is shown in Fig. 8.2.

November 16, 1990

Virus diarrhoea must be eradicated

Annual losses of 20-30,000 DKK

......We should in Denmark take the only reasonable decision to eradicate BVD......
....all animals must be tested and PI animals slaughtered....
Hereafter it must be anticipated that the disease dies out...

......It is important that costs for laboratory tests are reduced and that herds are certified and animals being tested before trade

November 30, 1990

BVD can not yet be eradicated

Irresponsible with a control program for BVD

......Before the eradication of Aujeszky's disease and IBR experiences with limited control programmes were obtained. For BVD we do not have such experiences......
......In general, BVD is spread from herd to herd by infected animals

But it can also be introduced by semen......It is not known if it is only the persistently infected animals that are responsible for continued transmission of infection

Figure 8.2. Translations of examples of headlines in a Danish farmers' newspaper November 1990.

The debate clearly showed that a lot of important information was available, but essential information was still missing. Table 8.6 shows examples of what was known and what information was lacking in the beginning of 1990s, just before the initiation of the Danish BVDV control and eradication programme.

Table 8.6. Examples of what was known and what information was still lacking in the beginning of 1990s just before the initiation of the Danish BVDV control and eradication programme.

1990		1990-1995
What did we know?	**What was lacking?**	**Closure of knowledge gap.**
Losses high in some herds	Average national losses	Estimated as GBP 13 million in 1993 (Houe et al., 1993)
Good laboratory tests on individual animals	Efficient and cheap tests at herd level	Spot sampling for use as herd tests developed (Houe, 1992)
PI animals important transmitters of infection	Practical importance of other transmission routes	Pilot project on the Island of Samsø (Bitsch and Rønsholt 1995)

References

Bitsch V, Rønsholt L, 1995. Control of bovine viral diarrhea virus infection without vaccines. Veterinary Clinics of North America. Food Animal Practice 11:627-640.

Houe H, 1992. Serological analysis of a small herd sample to predict presence or absence of animals persistently infected with bovine virus diarrhoea virus (BVDV) in dairy herds. Research in Veterinary Science 53: 320-323.

Houe H, Pedersen KM, Meyling A, 1993. A computerized spread sheet model for calculating total annual national losses due to bovine virus diarrhoea virus (BVDV) infection in dairy herds and sensitivity analysis of selected parameters. Proceedings of the Second Symposium on ruminant pestiviruses. 01-03 October 1992: 179-184.

Katholm J, Markmann C, 1994. BVD skal udryddes. Erfaringer med tankmælk-prøver og besætningssaneringer (BVD must be eradicated. Experiences with bulk milk testing and herd eradication, in Danish). Dansk Veterinærtidsskrift 77, 148-151.

9

Communication

9.1. Introduction

A structured programme includes a purpose and a goal, as well as a strategy to achieve this. This information (the purpose, the goal and the route to the goal) should also be communicated to the participants and stakeholders. Primary participants are most often the farmers supported by their herd health advisors, e.g. veterinary practitioners. A number of other parties may play minor but essential roles, and all stakeholders need to be identified and addressed at an appropriate level in order to make the programme successful. Establishing a communication plan could help serve this purpose. Some stakeholders should simply be informed, whereas others may have to participate in more elaborate education schemes depending on the complexity of the programme, and the specific role the stakeholder will play. The communication and education plan should be closely related to the purpose and timeframe of the programme, as well as the needs of the stakeholders. These needs may vary over time when the programme is in different phases. The current chapter focuses on elements in communication in the course of an infectious disease programme. Discussions and debates occurring prior to making the decision to eradicate are covered in Chapter 8.

9.2. Purpose, strategy and plan for communication

As in other projects, the purpose and goal of the programme are generally central to the establishment of the communication plan. However, the strategy for carrying out the programme is also important. There may be several ways to achieve the goal, but they may not be equally efficient, or feasible in all regions. It should be decided whether one or several strategies are recommended; and how to deal with alternative strategies, which are not officially part of the programme.

Perhaps one of the bigger risks is that some participants take elements of different strategies and create combinations that will not cover all the essential items to reach the goal (illustrated in Fig. 9.1). For example, one strategy for BVDV control could focus on detection and eradication of PI animals. Another strategy could be to keep the PI animals in order to continuously expose susceptible animals so that they have protective antibodies ('natural immunisation'). Both strategies may work well separately. However, if different farms vary in their approaches, those using the first strategy will create a population of completely naïve animals, and therefore a major risk of losses if mixed with animals from a population using the latter strategy.

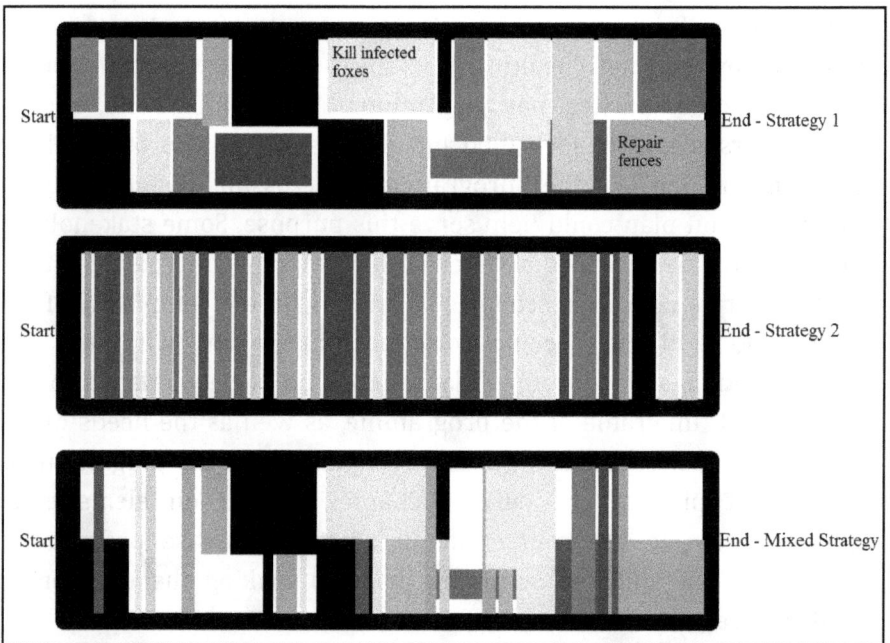

Figure 9.1. Possible effect of 'strategy mixing'. Three strategies to achieve a task are illustrated: Strategy 1, Strategy 2 and a mix of the two. Each element or task in the strategy is given by a specific box (e.g. 'Kill foxes'). Some tasks are small; some are large. Different operations are used to address an overall aim (indicated by the outer rectangle). Areas not covered in the strategy are shown in white. Strategies 1 and 2 may work equally well, whereas the mixed strategy has large uncovered areas, despite having the same average number of tasks as in Strategies 1 and 2. The result may well be that the goal is not achieved.

It is also possible that individual farmers find some elements of one strategy more inconvenient than similar elements of another strategy, and then choose the 'easier route'. However, such jumping between strategies may leave major areas uncovered, and the resulting overall strategy full of gaps (Fig. 9.1). Consequently, it may be beneficial to have only one strategy in a national/regional programme, in order to discourage stakeholders from being too creative and losing the battle against the infectious agent. A more specific example is provided in Fig. 9.2.

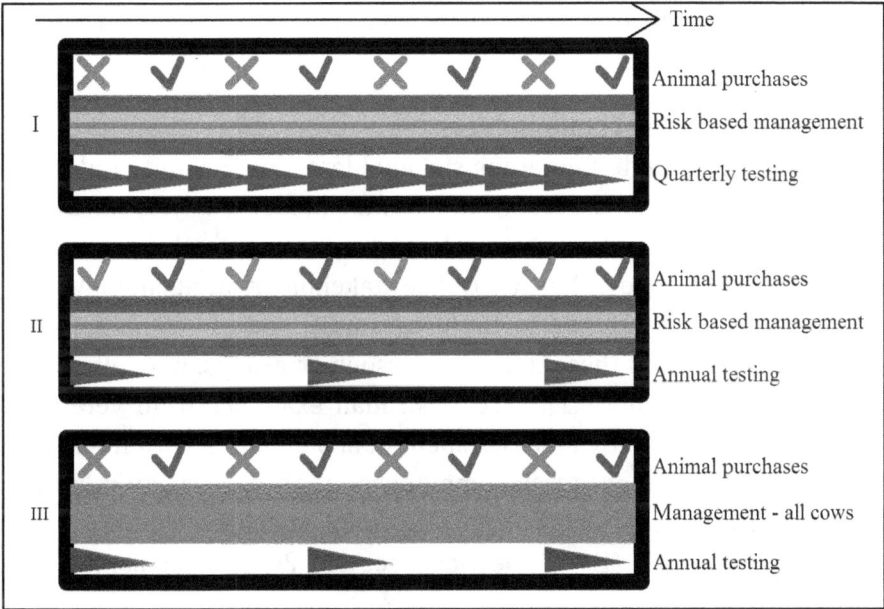

Figure 9.2. Three different strategies used to control MAP in a dairy herd. Strategy I is based on year-quarterly testing, which is a prerequisite for use of risk-based management. Strategy III includes only annual testing, but this strategy is not risk-based because specific management of all cows is carried out and is thus not dependent on the test-strategy. However, when mixing strategies I and III, with the resulting strategy II, a problem arises because valid test-results are not available for risk-based management of cows. Furthermore, in both strategies I and III, purchase of test-negative animals is possible (indicated by green √), but test-positives are not traded (red X). In strategy II, all animals are purchased irrespective of test-status (both

red and green √), while only test-negative animals can be purchased in Strategies I and III.

A primary benefit of a one-strategy approach is a simpler educational system; but the risk is that some people might still introduce alternative strategies, which could be merged with the original strategy creating inefficiency within the programme. Such situations should be covered in a communication plan. It is possible to make several strategies available simultaneously, but the associated educational and logistical requirements may prove more challenging. Essentially, the strategy should incorporate as many participants as possible while still retaining its efficiency.

9.3. Identification of stakeholders

Most projects include numerous stakeholders. Control and eradication programmes are no different, and a stakeholder analysis should be carried out to determine their role and relevance to the programme (Brugha and Varvasovszky, 2000). The stakeholders are generally those that affect, or are affected by the programme, and the communication plan should address these different persons or groups, who often have different roles (Table 9.1). Two Australian examples from veterinary medicine include firstly an assessment of stakeholders with interest in, or potential to influence risk communication on biosecurity related to small-scale pig production, and secondly management of equine influenza outbreak (Hernández-Jover et al., 2012; Schemann et al., 2014).

The list of stakeholders can be long, and it is not always the same groups of people who are relevant in specific programmes, or in all phases of a programme. The messages that should be conveyed to the different people or groups may also differ significantly, and appropriate language should be used accordingly (using scientific, farming or consumer terminology etc.). Farmers and herd health advisors are often the central stakeholders, but other people or groups may also play key roles. For example, bank managers may impact an individual herd's health programme by limiting the financial options to invest in farm housing, irrespective of whether the subsequent improvements to biosecurity will increase herd profitability in the long run. On the other hand, there are examples of banks that require improved biosecurity and demand effective disease control before investing in farms. Communication of such an aspect may well be included in a communication plan. Therefore, in summary, for each relevant stakeholder, the necessary information should be identified and communicated.

Table 9.1. List of potential stakeholders to consider including in a communication plan of a disease programme.

Stakeholder	Role, relevance or information needed
Farmer	Pays the costs; establishes barriers to reduce transmission; interprets test-results; gains from a successful programme.
Herd employees	Employees managing animals on a daily basis. Assist farmer in establishing biosecurity measures and interpreting test-results.
Farm employees	Employees not managing animals, but involved in crop production and thus feed management or with access to farm facilities, potentially spreading pathogen.
Herd health advisor	Advises on biosecurity measures; interprets test-results.
Other herd advisors	Advise on feeding, nutrition, housing etc. in the herd. This advice may work synergistically or antagonistically to the disease control efforts.
Other farm advisors	Advise on crops, economy and other factors which have direct impact on the management of the farm and thus indirect impact on management of the herd.
External technicians	Technicians with access to areas with animals (e.g. inseminators, milking equipment technicians and perhaps even milk truck drivers).
Processing plant workers	Workers at processing plants, such as milk collection centres and slaughterhouses, where the animal products may have to be managed in a specific way.

Farming industry	Policy makers often with interest in ensuring short and long-term farming profitability and maintaining a desirable industry image. May have a coordinating role.
Retail industry	Interested in safe food and good image of the food sold.
Consumers	Have impact on the value of products, and may have to be informed about infection risks, both with and without the programme, in order to retain or increase product value.
Politicians	National or regional governmental decision makers.
Authorities	If they are involved in carrying out decisions.
Animal activists	Have an impact on the value of products, and may have to be informed about benefits of programme, e.g. reduced mortality.
Researchers	Perform research e.g. for development and assessment of tools to mitigate transmission and establish diagnoses.
Teachers and educators	Develop training material for courses and teach farmers, advisors etc. on elements relevant to control or eradication efforts.

9.4. Who communicates what?

The various types of stakeholders should not receive information from just one source. The purpose of the communication should be clear, and the communicator selected accordingly. Lobbyists should campaign, trained educators train, and so forth. Researchers should communicate with researchers, and perhaps train advisors; whereas advisors may often be better training farmers. The primary industries may be more familiar than researchers with the requirements of authorities, but may not always be regarded with the same level of trust on some issues. All these circumstances need to be considered.

9.5. Information to be communicated

The type and level of information required by different stakeholders will obviously differ. Farmers, their primary herd-associated employees, and herd health advisors should often have detailed information, for example:

- the purpose and benefits of a successful programme;
- the strategy and expected timescale to achieve success;
- the operational elements necessary to achieve success;
- how success is monitored;
- where information about the programme can be obtained.

Furthermore, the communication strategy should contain elements on:

- the start and expected timeframe of the programme;
- follow-up after the success of the programme; and
- ways to keep participants motivated over time.

Herd and farm advisors should be informed about the purpose and benefits of the programme, in order for them to understand the importance. Furthermore, they should recognise elements that are directly influenced by choices they may make, as in the following examples:

1) Housing experts involved in construction of new barns should be approached to ensure that appropriate between-group sectioning is included in order to reduce transmission of pathogens between groups of animals.
2) Nutritionists should know of foodstuffs that may affect the animals' ability to cope with the infection, and consequently nutritionists should be informed of such possible adverse effects in a programme. For example, MAP infections have anecdotally been considered to deteriorate when feeding sugar water and beets (*Beta vulgaris* var. *rapacea*). Even without evidence of whether the anecdote is true or not, a failure to deal with the information appropriately may cause disturbance to the programme.
3) Technicians operating on multiple farms should be informed of the risks in transmitting the pathogen via equipment, clothes etc., and possibly how to clean the equipment if needed.

Some of the necessary messages can be very brief and may be mounted on entrances to the farm or the herd, for example: 'wash and disinfect boots prior to entry'; others can be included in information leaflets. However, information for farmers and herd health advisors may be of such detail that it is better to develop actual teaching material and provide course-like training.

9.6. Educational efforts

Passive information is unlikely to be sufficient for farmers and advisors, and a communication plan should detail how the necessary information can be communicated, and should assert the need for continuing education. There are basically three tasks: 1) engaging the participants; 2) encouraging them to do the right things to control or eradicate the infection; and 3) maintaining their engagement with the programme until it is complete. The more complex the pathogenesis and transmission patterns (and thus the programme and strategy) are, the bigger the need for educational efforts. However, farmers and their advisors are very heterogeneous groups with a variable need for details and learning modes etc. Some require courses, whereas others just need the right information to be available. These varied needs have to be addressed. Development of teaching material that can be used directly in the advisory process may be useful, such as on-farm risk assessment tools in paper format (Goeldner et al., 2011) or online (e.g. www.myhealthyherd.co.uk). There is still a great need to develop learning tools for assessment of efficient biosecurity measures, but this aspect is a key element in the educational efforts. Another primary element to be covered in the education process is interpretation and use of diagnostic test-results. The tests used should be fit-for-purpose, and proper interpretation of the results is the last step in that process. All the steps laid out in Chapter 5 on diagnostic tests, and the test-result interpretation should be taught to herd health advisors and, to some extent, also farmers. Thereby, frustrations about unexpected results may be avoided. As an example, the Danish MAP control programme in 2009 included five different test-reports (Nielsen, 2009) to cover different aspects in communication of test-results: a) overview of summarised herd results over time; b) overview of results for each cow over time; c) results used for management of infection (see Fig. 7.2); d) list of recommendations for cow-culling; and e) a list of recommendations for calf-culling. Certain reports are useful to some groups of people, whilst other reports are more useful to other people. Some reports cover the details, while others provide overviews. Essentially, summary information should be available to those requesting it, and details to those requiring them. Taking the view that farmers do not need or appreciate details may cause frustration, because many farmers prefer to have these details and do understand the concepts of, for example, false-positive and false-negative, if these are explained properly.

9.7. Long-term communication – keeping the stakeholders motivated

Once the programme is running, it is important to keep farmers aware of the status in their own herd, in 'similar' or 'competing' herds, or perhaps in specific regions etc. A continuous focus is needed, and small unofficial competitions may keep farmers motivated and aware of the possible risks. For example, the owner of a BVD-free herd should be aware of the continued risk of importing infected animals. The owner of an MAP-infected herd should be aware that a control scheme may last almost a decade in his/her farm, but the efforts should be continued every day until success has been achieved. Progress in controlling the prevalence or incidence on the farm, or in cohorts of farms with similar characteristics (stratification by region, breed, herd size, management system etc.), may be used for such purposes. Scientific achievements of interest to the programme can be published in farmers' magazines. The same can be the case for farmers' 'inventions' of practical relevance, e.g. tips on how to store colostrum in a freezer, or how to carry a slippery newborn without being soaked, and without hurting the calf. There are several options, but the primary objective is to keep farmers motivated to continue or improve their efforts.

9.8. Methods of communication

Publication of information in leaflets, farmers' magazines, and on websites is an obvious way of communicating messages. However, information meetings, seminars and the like may be more efficient in the beginning of a programme, due to the possibility of interaction. Thereby, focus can more easily be directed to areas that may be relevant to the stakeholders, if those developing the programme have neglected important areas.

The means by which messages are communicated also vary. Hard facts such as prevalences, costs, and benefits may be best presented as numbers or graphs; whereas the effects of stakeholder actions or principles may be better visualised in other ways. For example, the management focus related to the control of *S.* Dublin can be visualised with the risk of transmission in different management areas (Fig. 9.3). The principles for management of MAP in the Danish control programme were illustrated to farmers as shown in Fig. 9.4. More severe methods such as providing public information about the individual herd may be used, for example information on *S.* Dublin status is publicly available for all cattle herds via the Central Husbandry Register at: https://chr.fvst.dk/

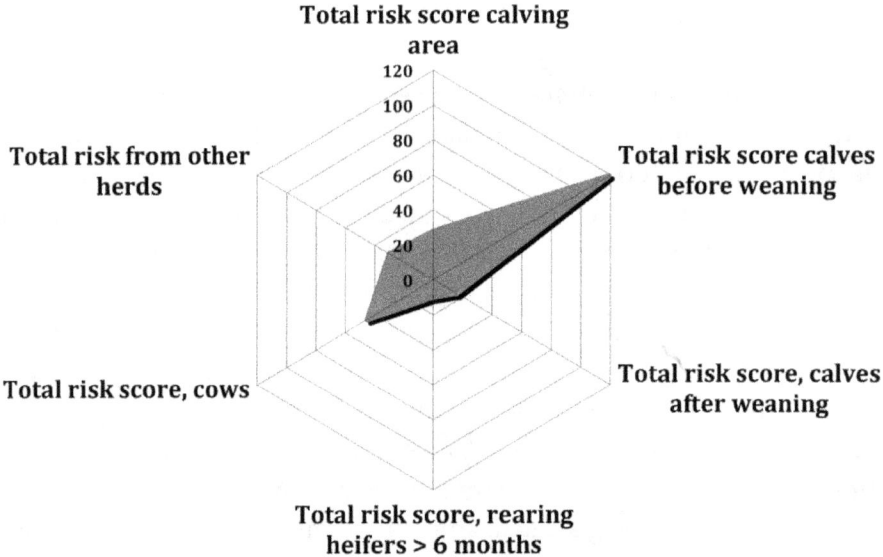

Figure 9.3. Risk scores for different management areas (MS Excel sheet supplied as supplementary material to Nielsen and Nielsen, 2012).

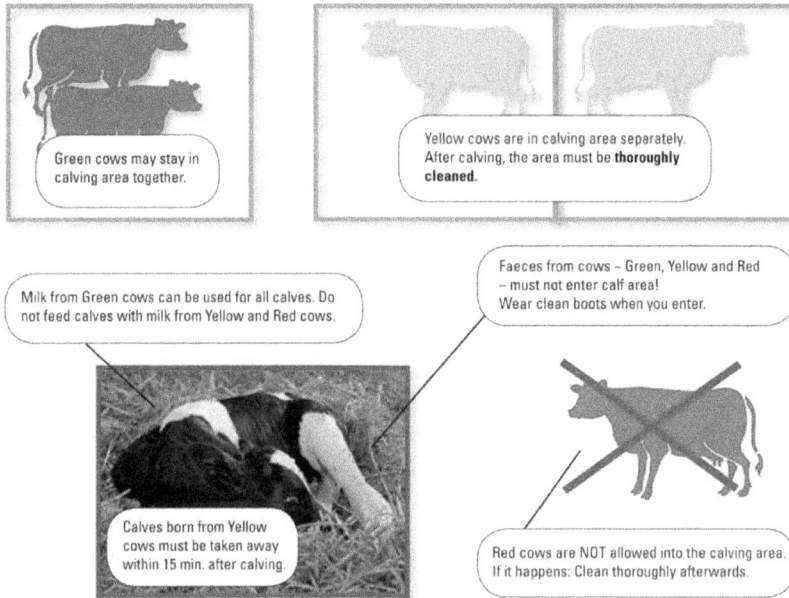

Figure 9.4. Extract from poster used by the Danish Cattle Federation to summarise the principles of the key management procedures to avoid within-herd transmission of MAP. This graphical presentation clearly points to the key focus area: calves before weaning.

Experience groups, where farmers meet on-farm to discuss various issues, are also an efficient way of interacting with colleagues for the purpose of discussing specific subjects. The 'stable school approach' (Vaarst, 2012) is a systematic approach that may be used for the purpose of learning while interacting. The principle in stable schools is that farmers are assembled in a farm to discuss a specific issue. A facilitator supports the discussion of the issue, but does not provide solutions on the issue. Possible solutions should come from the farmers in the group. For example, practical and effective biosecurity measures need to be identified and implemented to reduce transmission of MAP from dams to calves in the calving pen. How is this possible on the specific farm? Do the farmers determine that this is important, and can they identify solutions? The premise is that they know the options and limitations of the farm better than most people, and as a group they may see more solutions than as individuals. Therefore, they should be able to inspire each other to an extent that would be difficult for outsiders.

Again: there are various different modes of communication; some farmers have certain needs and preferences, and it is unlikely that all farmers and other stakeholders can be targeted with just one method of communicating the necessary information.

Some participants may be 'hard to reach' by information and communication alone; a 'carrot-and-stick' approach will most often be a necessity in the programme. Legislation may offer an option in such instances, but penalties or reduced prices are also commonly used e.g. a reduction in milk price associated with reduced milk quality due to high somatic cell counts. Examples of legislation to gradually tighten the grip on BVDV and *S.* Dublin first through surveillance, then control and later eradication are shown in Chapters 10 and 11.

References

Brugha R, Varvasovszky Z, 2000. Stakeholder analysis: a review. Health Policy Plan. 15:239-246.

Goeldner D, Patton E, Wheeler R, May GM, 2011. Handbook for Veterinarians and Producers. A guide for Johne's disease risk assessment and management plans for dairy herds. Available at: http://www.nd.gov/ndda/files/resource/DairyRiskAssessment1stYear 2011_0.pdf (cited 10 June 2013).

Hernández-Jover M, Gilmour J, Schembri N, Sysak T, Holyoake PK, Beilin R, Toribio JA, 2012. Use of stakeholder analysis to inform risk communication and extension strategies for improved biosecurity amongst small-scale pig producers. Preventive Veterinary Medicine 104:258-270.

Nielsen SS, 2009. Use of paratuberculosis tests in infected herds. Proceedings of the 2nd New Horizons in Johne's Disease Control workshop, University of Minneapolis, St. Paul, 09-10 August 2009, p. 32-39. Available at:

http://www.paratuberculosis.info/web/images/stories/pdfs/507.pdf (cited 10 June 2013).

Nielsen LR, Nielsen SS, 2012. A structured approach to control of *Salmonella* Dublin in 10 Danish dairy herds based on risk scoring and test-and-manage procedures. Food Research International 45: 1158-1165.

Schemann K, Gillespie JA, Toribio JA, Ward MP, Dhand NK 2014. Controlling equine influenza: Policy networks and decision-making during the 2007 Australian equine influenza outbreak. Transboundary and Emerging Diseases 61, 449-463.

Vaarst M, 2012. Reducing antibiotic usage in organic dairy farms - the stable school approach. Cattle Practice, 20, 157-161.

10

Follow-up investigations and adjustments of the eradication programme

10.1. Introduction

Even if a pilot study has been successful, there may still be unexpected elements to consider when the eradication campaign is run in a larger area, such as a country. If the disease control programme mitigates the impact of the main risk factors, then the relative importance of some of the remaining risk factors may be increased. For instance, if movement of cattle from infected to non-infected premises is a major risk factor, and this practice is stopped by programme restrictions, it may be that washing boots when entering a barn will then become a more important control effort in breaking transmission routes. It is also possible that important traits of either the infection or the production system may change, which could then impact the performance of the applied tests. For instance, when herds become larger, the sensitivity (Se) of bulk tank milk (BTM) testing may be reduced. This chapter emphasises the importance of systematically collecting and addressing all experiences obtained during the eradication phase. Furthermore, reduced incidence of infection as well as other changes may require some elements of the programme are amended, for example changes in the test-strategy and use of diagnostic techniques with features differing from those used in the high prevalence situations.

10.2. Identifying explanations for reinfections

During the eradication phase, herds are systematically classified as either infected or non-infected. This regular testing means that in many herds, detection of an infected animal can be considered a 'new' infection from an outside source, and not simply from one that has been hitherto undetected in the herd. This provides a good opportunity to study the possible outside sources of the infection. For example, in order to understand reasons for BVDV reinfection of Danish herds, an explorative follow-up study was made in recently infected herds, previously proven to be BVDV-free in the programme. Among 204 previously BVDV-free Danish dairy herds that became infected from 1997 to 1998, 67 (33% of the herds) were thoroughly investigated for possible reasons for reinfection. The most obvious circumstances to explain these reinfections among the 67 studied herds included: purchase of pregnant animals delivering PI animals (28%), PI animals on neighbouring pastures (36%), animals on common pasture (7%) and PI animals in neighbouring farm houses (3%). In the remaining 25% of the herds, no obvious explanation for infection could be identified (Bitsch et al., 2000). This type of study would not be feasible in a population with endemic infection at a high prevalence level and with no control program, as reinfections cannot be distinguished from continuous infections within the herds.

The follow-up studies showed that there were several aspects of biosecurity that could be improved, and that it might be important to gain a clearer understanding of farmers' motivation and reluctance to implement different biosecurity measures. A consequence of such follow-up studies may be that current legislation needs to be tightened (see next section). In addition, subtyping of pathogen strains can be an important means of tracing possible sources for new infections (Uttenthal et al., 2005).

10.3. Adjusting legislation during the eradication phase

From 1996 to 2006, ten ministerial orders were issued in Denmark to support eradication and minimise the spread of BVDV (Table 10.1). During these years, many biosecurity measures were included in the legislation. These had particular focus on avoiding contact with BVDV carrier animals. This control element was included to a very different extent in different ministerial orders: first by not allowing PI animals on pasture; later by ordering for them to be slaughtered or brought to an incinerating plant; and ultimately demanding that they be isolated or killed on the farm (Table 10.1).

Table 10.1. Key control elements included in Danish legislation during the BVDV eradication programme

Ministerial order no. and year / Control elements			1 96	2 96	3 97	4 99	5 99	6 01	7 02	8 04	9 04	10 06
Biosecurity of animal movements	Certificate before movement		X	X	X							
	Certificate dep. on herd status					X	X	X	X	X	X	
	Certificate not required											X
Biosecurity and elimination strategy of identified PI animals	Keep PI animals from pasture		X	X	X							
	Slaughter PI (or send to incinerating plant)					X	X	X				
	Isolate PI animals								X	X	X	X
	Kill or slaughter PI animals on farm										X	X
Systematic test-and-elimination strategy	Clarification of herd status	Owner	X	X	X	X	X	X	X			
		Dairy or abattoir								X	X	X
	Follow up	Test for PI							X	X		
		Action plan to eliminate								X	X	X
	Continued monitoring	Owner		X	X	X	X	X	X			
		Dairy or abattoir								X	X	X
Additional administrative reinforcements	Report to CHR database					X	X	X	X	X	X	X
	Notifiable		X	X	X	X	X	X	X	X	X	X
	Inform visitors and neighbours		X	X	X	X	X	X	X	X	X	X

The risk of transmission via livestock was initially addressed on individual animal level, where diagnostic tests were used as a basis to issue certificates before movement. Later, when freedom from infection could be accurately determined at herd level, the demands for individual certificates were replaced by declaration of herd status. Biosecurity measures that had less evidence of importance in literature (such as indirect transmission by utensils and clothing) were included in legislation to a lesser extent. Due to changing situations over the years, there have been examples of control elements for which it was necessary to heighten the demands; but conversely also control elements for which procedures could become more flexible.

There may also be a need to demonstrate compliance with legislation. This was seen in the BVDV eradication programme, where lawsuits resulted in court orders demanding non-compliant farmers to pay for any losses incurred by other farms that had been caused by their infected herds.

10.4. Change in test-strategy – change in sensitivity and specificity

Although it is often said that the diagnostic sensitivity (Se) and specificity (Sp) of tests at an individual animal level are independent of the prevalence, this is not always the case in practice. This may be due to: a) a reduction in the disease severity distribution resulting in reduced Se (Ransohoff and Feinstein, 1978); and b) atypical cases being more difficult to detect and therefore tending to remain until the later stages.

At herd level, considerable changes can be seen in herd Se (HSe) and herd Sp (HSp) along with the decline in the number of infected animals. For example, in the early stages of BVDV eradication in specific herds, the cleared herds would still have many antibody carriers, and monitoring for freedom of infection could only be done by testing young animals for antibodies. However, in later stages in these herds, it was possible to monitor by only testing BTM (see Chapter 11.2.9), i.e. the Sp (and hence positive predictive value) of BTM testing was becoming much higher. At an even later stage, the positive predictive value (PPV) declined again, following the general rule that PPV declines along with a declining prevalence. Thus in naïve populations, a greater number of false positives can be expected. However, all test positive results must still be taken seriously and follow-up investigations made, so that a positive test can be either confirmed or ruled out.

Over time, there may also be variations among other factors affecting test performance. For example in Denmark, the herd size increased considerably during the first years of the eradication programme. As in this example, the antibodies will undergo a higher dilution in BTM, which will affect the HSe of the BTM test.

A change from testing individual animals to BTM testing might be desirable, due to a reduction in costs. However, it may not always be possible. For example, farmers began requesting that BTM testing was used 5-6 years after the Danish MAP programme started in 2006, even though this type of testing was not a logical option based on knowledge of the infection dynamics. Whilst BVDV infections often lead to a high within-herd prevalence of cows with antibodies, MAP infections usually result in a low within-herd antibody prevalence. Development of the antibody response usually only occurs in late-stage infection and in older animals; not in the young animals with latent infection. Consequently, few latent infections could be present without the disease being detectable. However, this argument was not generally accepted, so data had to be collected to support it (Nielsen and Toft, 2014). This demonstrates that in such cases, data may be better in supporting the argument than knowledge transferred from other infections.

10.5. Transition from control and eradication to surveillance for documentation of freedom and early detection of new infections

A change in the test-strategy is usually also related to changes in the overall focus or purpose of the programme, e.g. a change from control and eradication to surveillance, as the infection is gradually becoming exotic. Although exotic infections are beyond the scope of this book, 'the transition period' from endemic to exotic diseases will be covered. Once an area or country has obtained freedom from a specific disease, the focus of the test-strategy changes from classifying herds into infected or non-infected, to continued documentation of freedom, and also to early detection of potential new introductions of infection.

There may be variation in how early different laboratory techniques can detect a new infection, resulting in longer detection times in some situations. To improve early detection of BVDV infections, it has been recommended that the antigen ELISA be replaced with PCR techniques as these can also detect viruses in antibody-positive calves (Uttenthal et al., 2005).

A way to improve early detection (and monitoring and surveillance in general) is the use of sentinel herds (McCluskey, 2003). In general, the principle of sentinel surveillance is to target herds or areas with higher probabilities of infection, for example herds with naïve animals that are located in areas known to be at high risk of introduction of new infections, e.g. close to borders to countries with endemic infection. Repeated testing of these animals at certain intervals increases the probability of early detection. Quantitative risk assessment can be used to identify areas with higher risk of infection, and has been used, for example, to identify areas in Spain with higher risk of introduction of foot-and-mouth disease (Martínez-López et al., 2008). When formulating plans for early detection, it must also be considered whether initial detection is more likely to be made by clinical observation (as with foot-and-mouth disease), or whether it is likely that the infection can be introduced without any obvious clinical signs (as with BVDV infection). In the former case, passive surveillance based on reporting of clinical suspicions may be adequate.

10.6. Preparedness in 'peacetime'
When a disease has been eradicated for many years, there may be a tendency at many levels to forget its importance. Teachers at universities may tend to focus more on the endemic diseases present in the country, and veterinary practitioners may be less aware of the infection over time. Therefore, it is important that the disease becomes part of the contingency planning for exotic diseases, and that continued awareness and preparedness is maintained. The preparedness includes close monitoring of the international disease situation, in particular in neighbouring countries. For some diseases, there are international standards provided by OIE for declaration of freedom. But for other diseases, there are no standards and the surveillance system decided upon can vary between individual countries and regions (Doherr et al., 2003). This can make the judgement of current threat quite complicated.

References

Bitsch V, Hansen K-EL, Rønsholt L, 2000. Experiences from the Danish programme for eradication of bovine virus diarrhoea (BVD) 1994–1998 with special reference to legislation and causes of infection. Veterinary Microbiology 77: 137-143.

Doherr MG, Audigé L, Salman MD, Gardner IA, 2003. Use of animal monitoring and surveillance systems when the frequency of health-related events is near zero. *In* (Salman MD, *ed.*): Animal Disease Surveillance and Survey Systems. Methods and Applications. Blackwell Publishing, Ames, Iowa, ISBN 0-8138-1031-0.

Houe H, Baker JC, Maes RK, Ruegg PL, Lloyd JW, 1995. Application of antibody titers against bovine viral diarrhea virus (BVDV) as a measure to detect herds with cattle persistently infected with BVDV. Journal of Veterinary Diagnostic Investigation 7: 327-332.

Martínez-López, B., Perez, A.M., De la Torre, A., Zánchez-Vizcaíno Rodriguez JM, 2008. Quantitative risk assessment of foot-and-mouth disease introduction into Spain via importation of live animals. Preventive Veterinary Medicine 86: 43-56.

McCluskey BJ, 2003. Use of sentinel herds in monitoring and surveillance systems. *In* (Salman MD. *ed.*): Animal Disease Surveillance and Survey Systems. Methods and Applications. Blackwell Publishing, Ames, Iowa, ISBN 0-8138-1031-0.

Nielsen SS, Toft N, 2014. Bulk tank milk ELISA for detection of antibodies to *Mycobacterium avium* subsp. *paratuberculosis*: Correlation between repeated tests and within-herd antibody-prevalence. Preventive Veterinary Medicine 113: 96-102.

Ransohoff DF, Feinstein AR, 1978. Problems of spectrum and bias in evaluating the efficacy of diagnostic tests. New England Journal of Medicine 299:926-930.

Uttenthal Å, Stadejek T, Nylin B, 2005. Genetic diversity of bovine viral diarrhoea viruses (BVDV) in Denmark during a 10-year eradication period. Acta Pathologica Microbiologica et Immunologica Scandinavica 113: 536-541.

11

Description of example diseases and their related control and eradication programmes in Denmark

11.1. Introduction
The following chapter provides the main facts and features for each of the three diseases used as the primary examples in this book. Emphasis is on providing the reader with an understanding of the features of the disease that are of importance in different elements of control and eradication. For a more comprehensive understanding of the diseases themselves, the reader is referred to other literature.

11.2. Bovine virus diarrhoea
11.2.1. Introduction

The first clinical description of bovine virus diarrhoea (BVD) was presented in 1946 in the USA (Olafson et al., 1946), and was characterised principally by salivation, diarrhoea and erosions in the oral cavity, oesophagus and gastrointestinal tract. The condition had high morbidity, but low mortality. A few years later, the first description of 'mucosal disease' appeared (Ramsey and Chivers, 1953). This was a condition with similar but more severe clinical signs, and almost all affected animals were young stock (YS). Furthermore, the morbidity was low and the lethality (case fatality) was high. Later, after demonstrating the viral aetiology, it became clear that 'bovine virus diarrhoea virus' (BVDV) was the cause of both of these two clinically distinct disease expressions, and that the virus could cause a number of additional clinical manifestations. Thus, in infected herds, there could be problems with repeat breeding, abortions, high neonatal mortality, congenital defects and reduced growth rate among calves.

One of the main challenges of the infection was to understand how the same pathogen could result in two clinically different disease expressions. The underlying explanation was given by elucidating the pathogenesis, and some major breakthroughs occurred in the 1980s, laying the grounds for both developing test-strategies and instigating relevant biosecurity. The clinical manifestations resulted in severe losses to the farmers. Therefore, strong financial incentives for a control programme were present early on. As mentioned in Chapter 8, one of the main concerns about deciding on a control and eradication programme was the presence of a large number of possible transmission routes, of which the practical importance had to be determined before a programme could be initiated on a larger scale. All these aspects will therefore be described below, concluding with a presentation of the Danish BVDV control and eradication programme.

11.2.2. The aetiological agent, bovine virus diarrhoea virus

The virus BVDV belongs to the genus pestivirus in the family Flaviviridae (OIE, 2004). The virus can appear as one of two different biotypes, the cytopathic (CP) and the non-cytopathic (NCP) biotype, which either as the NCP alone or as the two biotypes in combination is essential for the pathogenesis and different clinical manifestations of infection (see later). Furthermore, the viruses are categorised in two main genotypes, namely BVDV Type 1 and BVDV Type 2. Recently, an atypical BVDV Type 3 has also been described. Additionally, the different types are characterised by a number of sub-groups showing some antigenic diversity (Ridpath, 2010). The BVDV types show some variation in virulence, in that BVDV Type 2 typically has caused more severe clinical signs including haemorrhages and thrombocytopenia.

The survival of the virus in the environment is highly dependent on the temperature. At 20°C, BVDV was inactivated after 3 days, whereas at 35°C survival was as short as 4 hours, and at 5°C inactivation has been shown to occur after 3 weeks (Bøttner & Belsham, 2012). Compared with other viruses in the Flaviridae family, pestivirus is resistant to inactivation by low pH, but the lipid envelope of the virus makes it susceptible to inactivation by organic solvents and detergents (Ridpath, 2010). For example, aromatic compounds can eliminate BVDV infections in foetal cells (Givens et al., 2004).

11.2.3. Pathogenesis

Postnatal infection is usually via the oronasal route, followed by viral replication in the respiratory tract. After a few days, the infection is followed by viraemia, which typically lasts 2-3 weeks. Hereafter, a slow rise in antibody level develops over several weeks. Following natural infection, antibodies are long lasting and often lifelong. This part of the pathogenesis is usually referred to as transient or acute infection of immunocompetent animals.

The main feature of the pathogenesis of BVDV infection is that during transient infection, the virus will cross the placenta and infect the foetus. If the foetus is infected during the first 3-4 months of gestation, it will develop immunotolerance (McClurkin et al., 1984). If not aborted, these foetuses are later born as persistently infected (PI) animals and will have a high and lifelong viraemia. The persistent infection is induced by the non-cytopathegenic strain of the virus. If the PI calf is later infected by a cytopathogenic strain (either by mutation of the existing strain or by infection from outside), this will often result in the clinical condition mucosal disease (Bolin et al., 1985; Brownlie et al., 1984).

In addition to fatality due to mucosal disease, the PI animals may also show a variety of clinical signs such as growth retardation, ill-thrift and increased susceptibility to other infections. However, a number of PI animals can remain clinically normal and develop into apparently healthy adult cows (Houe, 1992; 1993). Calves born to PI animals will always be PI animals themselves.

11.2.4. Diagnosis

There are many specific stages of infection that can be diagnosed by different laboratory techniques (reviewed in Dubovi, 2013; Goyal, 2005; Saliki & Dubovi, 2004; Sandvik, 2005):

a) Animals undergoing transient infection with low-grade viraemia for 1-2 weeks.
b) Immune animals with a previous transient infection (often with high and lifelong antibodies).

c) Calves that are born immunocompetent, but are antibody-positive for some months due to colostrum uptake.

d) Calves that are born PI, but are antibody-positive for some weeks due to colostrum uptake.

e) Calves that are born PI, with lifelong viraemia persisting after the colostral antibodies have waned.

f) Totally naïve (susceptible) animals that are both antibody and virus-negative.

Due to the long and stable condition of stages b) and e) in particular, good laboratory tests with high sensitivity (Se) and specificity (Sp) for detection of antibodies and virus in these two conditions have been fundamental in the BVDV control and eradication programmes.

Antibodies can be detected by different techniques such as virus neutralisation tests and different types of ELISAs. Generally, the Se and Sp for detection of antibodies in the individual animal is very high (more than 95%). For example, a Se of 96.5% and Sp of 97.5% for the Danish blocking ELISA (evaluated using a serum neutralisation test) were reported by Rønsholt et al. (1997). The virus isolation test has been used as the reference test for detection of virus, but different ELISAs are also widely used here. Compared to virus isolation, the blocking ELISA has high Se and Sp; for example, a Se of 97.9% and Sp of 99.5% were reported by Rønsholt et al (1997).

Therefore, for the two main categories of infected animals (i.e. the ones which have experienced transient infection more than some weeks ago, and the ones that are PI) the diagnostic techniques provide high Se and Sp.

Concerning infection stage a) above, it should be noted that as the transiently infected animals are typically viraemic for only 1-2 weeks, they are rarely detected. But due to the short viraemic phase in transiently infected animals, proof of persistent infection can only be reached by testing the animal twice at least 2 weeks apart, and if both tests are virus-positive.

Regarding detection of PI animals, virus detection may be hampered for some weeks due to the presence of colostral antibodies, as described in stage d. However, the use of immunohistochemical analysis on skin biopsy (e.g. ear notch samples) can still detect the virus despite the presence of colostral antibodies. PCR analysis can also be used, and this technique has high Se in specimens with low quantities of virus, and hence is suitable in suspected PI animals with colostral antibodies (Uttenthal et al., 2005).

11.2.5. Transmission

Cattle are the main source of the infection. Other species including small ruminants, pigs and many species of wild animal may be infected, but they do not have major practical importance in a control programme. Thus, cattle are considered the most relevant species with regards to maintaining the infection in an area and hence are the target species in a control programme.

Transmission can occur by direct contact between acutely or PI and susceptible animals. Infection via semen and embryos is also possible, if preventive actions are not taken. The infection is always transmitted much more efficiently from PI animals. This has been demonstrated in both experimental and observational studies (Houe and Meyling, 1991; Niskanen et al., 1996; Tråvén et al., 1991). Airborne transmission over short distances is possible. For example, airborne transmission via a 1.4m long tube was demonstrated by Mars et al., (1999). However, it is not clear precisely how far the virus can be transmitted by airborne transmission.

Several experimental studies have shown the possibility of indirect vehicle or vector transmission, e.g. by needles and nose tongs (Gunn, 1993), rectal gloves (Lang-Ree et al., 1994) and blood-feeding flies (Tarry et al., 1991). As many of these findings are based on experimental studies, their practical importance may be difficult to determine. However, reusing needles, medicine bottles and contaminated vaccines has been shown to cause transmission in the field (Barkema et al., 2001; Katholm and Houe, 2006; Løken et al., 1991; Valle et al., 1999).

11.2.6. Epidemiology

Before the first control programmes were initiated in the 1990s, BVDV infection occurred in all cattle populations studied throughout the world. A typical pattern in many countries was a high level endemic occurrence with PI animals in approximately 50% of the herds and presence of antibody carriers in almost all herds (Houe, 2005). The overall prevalence of PI animals in these regions was around 1-2%, and the prevalence of antibody carriers more than 60%. The large discrepancy between occurrence of antibody carriers and PI animals is due to the fact that a transiently infected cow needs to be in the first trimester of pregnancy in order to produce a PI calf. After the first infection, foetuses in following pregnancies would be protected. Although the overall prevalence of PI animals is relatively low in the overall population, they still occur in a considerable number of herds and thus maintain the infection in the area.

A typical pattern of transmission within the herd is that a limited number of cows undergo transient infection, after which the transmission stops. However, a number of PI-foetuses result from the transient infection, which will start to infect the remaining susceptible animals in the herd soon after they are born. A few months after the birth of the first PI animal, most other animals in the herd will become antibody-positive (Houe, 1993). In some countries (e.g. the US), the prevalence of PI animals is much lower than the previously mentioned 1-2%, and different transmission patterns within herds are sometimes seen. Such differences may be due to differences in demographic factors such as cattle density in the area, and whether animals within the farm are housed in close vicinity or in separated epidemiological units.

11.2.7. Effects of BVDV infection

Several different production losses can follow BVDV infections. Although the transient infection is often subclinical, some virulent strains, in particular among Type 2, have caused very high mortality rates (Carman et al., 1998). The general immunosuppression that follows transient infection has been shown to increase the risk of a number of other diseases. Transient infection may also be followed by reduced milk production and higher somatic cell count. In particular, reproductive losses are seen including decreased conception rate, abortions, congenital defects and high neonatal mortality. Among the PI animals that survive the neonatal period, many will be ill-thriven and considerably smaller than calves of the same age. Most PI calves will die or be culled before the age of 2 years. Some PI animals may appear clinically normal, reach adulthood and even have their own calves. Such calves from PI dams will always be PI themselves. Importantly, these clinically normal PI animals have huge implications for continued transmission of infection as they remain undetected and continuously excrete high amounts of virus.

Due to variation in virulence and the variation in gestational stages at the time of infection, the clinical manifestations can vary substantially between herd outbreaks. As mentioned in Chapter 3, the financial losses at herd level can vary substantially, e.g. from approximately EUR 20 to 600 per cow present in a herd, and the average losses per cow at the national level have been estimated at EUR 15 to 20 in some countries (Saatkamp et al., 2006). Although, these figures have high degree of uncertainty, it is still clear from early on that an efficient programme would be highly cost-effective.

In addition to the financial losses, mucosal disease causes a great deal of pain to the animal, adding to the importance of the infection. Yet the economic importance has still been the strongest motivator for initiating control programmes.

11.2.8. BVDV control and eradication

In the 1990s, the first BVDV control and eradication campaigns were introduced in the Scandinavian countries (Lindberg and Alenius, 1999). It took them approximately 10 years to reach the final stages of eradication and they have managed to stay free (or almost free) of infection in the years following eradication (Ståhl and Alenius, 2012). Control programmes have now also been initiated in a number of other European countries including Switzerland, Austria and Germany (Moennig et al., 2005; Presi et al., 2011; Rossmanith et al., 2010).

The overall considerations on selecting a control strategy or eradication programme have also been a hot topic in relation to BVDV. In many countries, the use of BVDV vaccines has been (and remains) widespread. Recently, it has been recommended that vaccination could be combined with a systematic test-strategy within an eradication programme, rather than viewing the two approaches as conflicting (Moennig et al., 2005).

11.2.9. The Danish BVDV control and eradication programme

A Danish control and eradication programme was launched on a voluntary basis in 1994 (Bitsch et al., 2000). Initially, the term 'control and eradication programme' was used, but later it was changed to 'eradication programme'.

From the beginning of the 1990s (i.e. in the years before the initiation of the programme), it became clear that BVDV infection was widespread in Danish cattle farms in that approximately half of the herds had PI animals (Houe, 1996; Houe and Meyling 1991). In some herds, the infection caused devastating losses to the farmer (See Fig. 11.2.1).

September 27, 1991

Cattle disease had shock course

Family loses 200,000 DKK due to attack from virus diarrhoea

......The family is in a shock condition...... ....During 5 months they have lost 5 cows due to BVD and 21 unborn calves due to abortion 5-6 months in gestation.... ...

......The milk yield has dropped approximately 20 %. ....The losses are estimated to be around 200,000 including 100,000 DKK due to loss in milk production.....

...... Purchased heifers were carriers with BVDV...... ....The buyers of animals to the farm should obtain guarantee that the purchased animals are not carriers of the virus.

Figure 11.2.1. Newspaper headline on BVDV. Translation from a Danish Farmers' newspaper, September 1991.

Such examples emphasised the need to take some form of action to control the disease. The motivation was further strengthened by the estimation of national economic losses at GBP 13 million, per million calving (Houe et al., 1993).

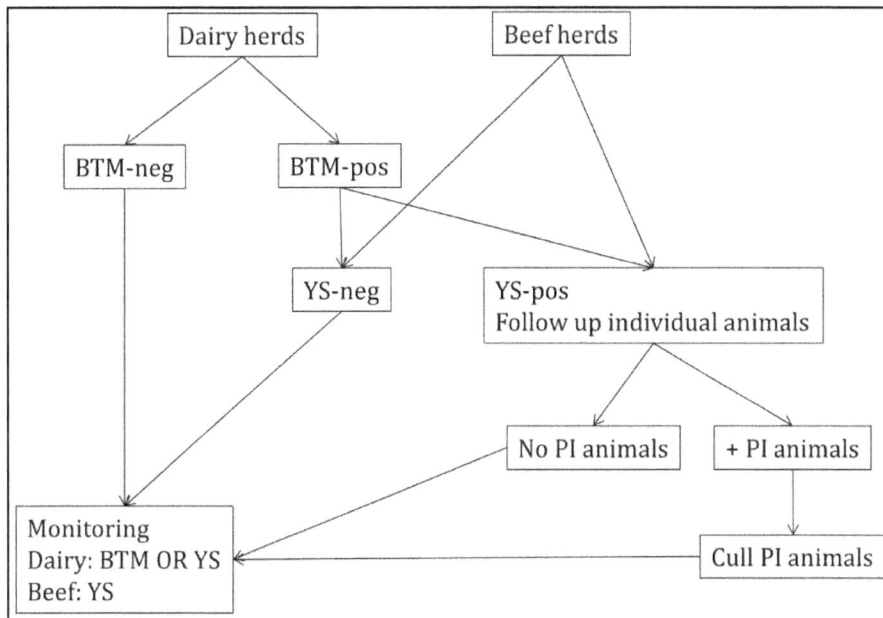

Figure 11.2.2. Decision tree for the test-strategy in the Danish BVDV and eradication programme. BTM: Bulk tank milk; YS: Young stock. The test-strategy contains the following steps and decisions:

a) Classification of herd infection status (herds with no or limited information of prior infection): Testing BTM in dairy herds or spot test of a few (YS) in beef herds.

b) Dairy herds that are BTM negative go directly to continued monitoring. In dairy herds with positive BTM, a spot sample of a few YS are tested.

c) Dairy and beef herds where animals in YS sample are negative go to monitoring.

d) In herds with AB positive YS, follow-up testing is performed to identify individual PI animals.

e) If no PI animals are identified, the herd goes to continued monitoring.

f) If PI animals are identified they are culled and after a follow-up period of identifying additional PI animals, the herd goes to continued monitoring.

g) Monitoring usually consists of testing BTM in dairy herds. In dairy herds that have recently been cleared, as well as in beef herds, monitoring is done by test of a spot sample of YS.

It soon became clear that the biosecurity measures in the programme should mainly focus on targeting specific infection stages of the animals, whereas external survival of the virus was less important. Although both transiently and persistently infected animals are infectious, it was the identification and removal of the PI animals in particular that was deemed crucial to the programme. Therefore, a systematic test-strategy beginning with the least costly test was established (Fig. 11.2.2).

Due to the widespread occurrence of the infection, it was decided to evaluate the potential for wide-scale eradication using a pilot project on the Island of Samsø (with approximately 110 producers). Furthermore, there was a desire to assess the practical suitability of the test-strategies outlined in Fig. 11.2.2 (see also Chapter 6). In particular, the systematic test and elimination strategy at the herd level was extremely cost-effective, and was therefore a key component of the programme. Soon after the conclusion of the pilot projects, the decision to initiate a general control and eradication programme was taken by the Danish cattle industry (Bitsch and Rønsholt, 1995).

The farmers' own organisations allocated resources for the organisation of the programme, and communicated general information about the disease, as well as methods for control and eradication, in order to motivate farmers from the very early stages. One of the more direct methods used to engage farmers was the distribution of information regarding the antibody level in their BTM.

To support the follow-up of the BVDV programme, the first ministerial order was issued in 1996. This stipulated that animals required a specific BVDV health certificate to be awarded before being moved to other herds and to common pastures. In addition, PI animals should be kept away from pastures, and owners of infected herds should inform neighbours and visitors about their infection status. Over the next 10 years, nine additional BVDV ministerial orders were issued to make the programme more efficient (see Chapter 10).

At the start of the programme in 1994, it was estimated that 39% of the dairy herds had PI animals. In 1999, 9% of the dairy herds and 5% of the beef herds had PI animals (Bitsch et al., 2000). The number of infected herds in Denmark between the year 2000 and the point at which the infection was practically eradicated is shown in Fig. 11.2.3. During the eradication phase, a number of infection-free herds became infected (see Chapter 10), but the programme was sufficiently effective as to identify and clear such herds.

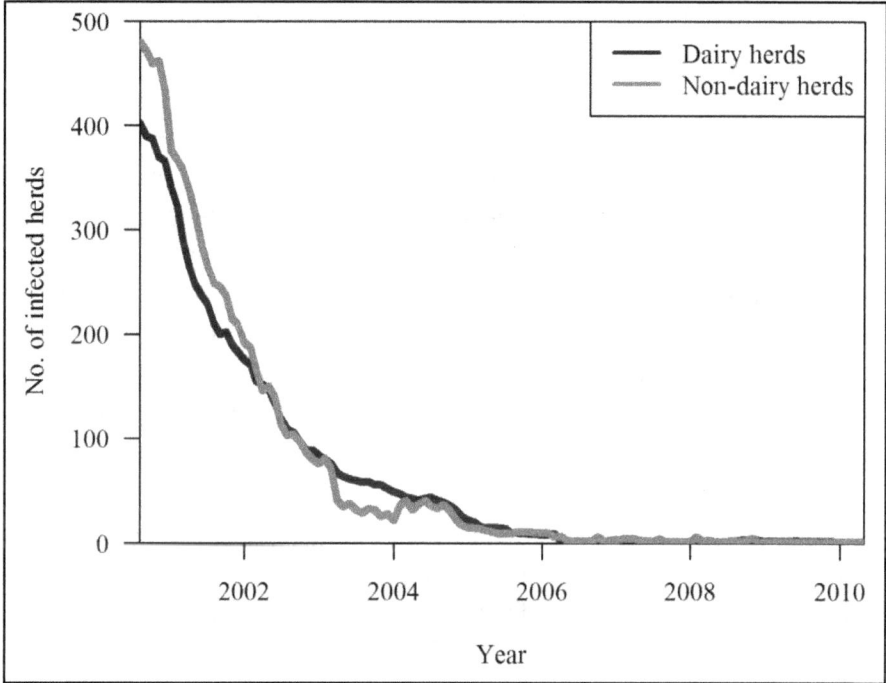

Figure 11.2.3. Decline in the number of BVDV infected herds during the final years of the BVDV eradication programme in Denmark. For comparison, the total numbers of dairy and non-dairy herds in the year 2000 were approximately 10,500 and 21,500 respectively, and these numbers were reduced to 3,478 dairy herds and 14,583 non-dairy herds in July 2014.

11.3. *Salmonella* Dublin

<u>11.3.1. Introduction</u>

Salmonella enterica subsp. *enterica* serovar Dublin (*S.* Dublin) is a bacterium that is host-adapted to cattle. Historical reports of salmonellosis in cattle originate back to the year 1865, when 'calf paratyphoid' outbreaks were described in Germany, the Netherlands and Denmark. Exactly which serotype caused these outbreaks is unknown (Wray and Davies, 2000). In 1891, C.O. Jensen described the bacteria '*Bacillus paracoli*' that was responsible for these outbreaks, and he reproduced the disease experimentally in calves (Jensen, 1891). He described it as a very pathogenic and invasive variant of other rod-shaped enteric bacteria (most likely *Escherichia coli*), which were also found in healthy animals. In the early 1900s, there were outbreaks in both adult cattle and young animals in Europe and the USA. In the outbreak reports, the bacteria were described in more detail, though the nomenclature was still confusing. This was improved by the extensive work of F. Kauffmann and B. White, which lead to description of a large number of salmonella serotypes often named after the geographical location where the first strain was isolated (Grimont et al., 2000). The isolation of similar bacteria from a human case in Dublin, Ireland, was reported in 1926 (Pesch, 1926). At first it was thought to be *Salmonella* Enteritidis. However in 1939 after further analysis, it was determined to be an individual serotype and was named after the first geographical location of isolation, hence the name *S.* Dublin.

S. Dublin is associated with increased morbidity, mortality and production losses including reduced milk yield in many infected cattle herds (Nielsen et al., 2013). Outbreaks in other species (e.g. mink and sheep) also occur. However, the source can usually be traced back to cattle, for example through slaughterhouse waste or contact to cattle or cattle manure. Moreover, *S.* Dublin is zoonotic and in human patients can lead to a severe infection characterised by septicaemia and a high fatality risk. Humans most frequently become infected through consumption of contaminated beef, but outbreaks have also been traced to products such as cheese and ice cream produced using unpasteurised milk, or where the pasteurisation process had failed (Maguire et al., 1992; Mateus et al., 2008).

A national strategy for control of *S.* Dublin in the Danish cattle population was developed in the early 2000s by the cattle industry and the veterinary authorities. In 2007 a national eradication programme was officially announced which aimed to reduce the national herd prevalence of *S.* Dublin to close to zero, and terminate spread of *S.* Dublin in the Danish cattle population.

The challenges associated with control and eradication efforts include: a) multiple infection stages with both subclinical as well as acute or chronic clinical disease expressions. Infections can be both active and latent, and can therefore presumably - although not necessarily - persist for a period of months to years; b) lack of understanding about the pathogenesis, in particular which factors determine the infection stages and the duration of infection that each individual will undergo upon exposure and infection; c) lack of sensitive diagnostic tests to detect infectious cattle; d) long survival in the environment; e) farmers lacking motivation due to variable clinical expression in infected herds and varying effects on farming profitability; and f) lack of effective or cost-effective vaccination strategies. These aspects along with transmission and epidemiology will therefore be described, before a presentation and discussion of elements of the Danish *S.* Dublin control and eradication programmes are covered.

11.3.2. The agent, *Salmonella enterica* subsp. *enterica* serovar Dublin (*S.* Dublin)

S. Dublin is one of more than 2,600 *Salmonella* serovars belonging to the genus *Salmonella* in the family Enterobactericeae. It is Gram-negative, oxidase-negative and rod-shaped. It is sensitive to most disinfectants, direct sunlight and to many types of antibiotics, although multidrug-resistant strains have been isolated from some beef and dairy sources. If surrounded by organic matter such as stored slurry, cattle manure and soil, it can survive for months or even years in the environment (Plym-Forshell and Ekesbo, 1996; Taylor and Burrows, 1971). Therefore environmental hygiene, including effective removal of faecal matter from the animals' immediate surroundings is an essential part of the control efforts. The survival of *S.* Dublin in slurry has been found to depend on temperature, pH, microflora, slurry treatment and storage conditions (Jones, 1976; Jones et al., 1977). Outside of the host, the bacteria can even multiply in warm and moist conditions, adding to the difficulty in controlling transmission via the environment (Wray and Davies, 2000). Although there are many different strains of *S.* Dublin with varying virulence, the serotype is characterised by few clonal lineages, and there is a large overlap in clonal lineages between strains isolated from different species, including humans (Olsen and Skov, 1994). This may indicate that there are only few common original sources, and it means that more discriminative methods (including full genome sequencing) are necessary to facilitate epidemiological investigations of transmission routes and sources of infection (Kjeldsen et al., 2014).

11.3.3. Pathogenesis

The mechanisms of host adaptation are not well understood, and invasiveness varies between the different *S.* Dublin strains. However, the fact that *S.* Dublin is host-adapted facilitates the control of the infection within the cattle sector. Uptake of *S.* Dublin is usually via the faecal-oral route. The bacteria can be ingested directly from faeces, contaminated feed, water, milk or the immediate environment. Upon ingestion the bacteria reach the gastrointestinal lumen, colonise and invade the gut epithelial cells as soon as 6 hours after uptake, and may be shed in faeces within 12-24 hours after exposure. Hence, *S.* Dublin is often a fast-spreading infection when it enters a naïve population. Acidic conditions in the gastrointestinal canal inhibit *S.* Dublin growth and colonisation, and gut motility reduces its ability to adhere to the intestinal epithelium. Furthermore, the bacteria are inactivated by local non-specific, cell-mediated and humoral immune responses in the gut. Therefore in physiologically stable cattle the susceptibility to *S.* Dublin decreases with age. However, sufficiently large doses can affect cattle of all ages, and co-infections, illness or other types of stressors such as transportation or crowded barns can reduce resistance to the bacteria. Cell-mediated immunity is more important for the protection of cattle against *S.* Dublin than the humoral immunity. Serum antibodies do not provide sufficient immunity for the animal against these highly invasive and intracellular bacteria. However, antibodies directed against *S.* Dublin are useful for diagnostics, as described below.

It is thought that *S.* Dublin can lead to several different infection stages in cattle. Calves are usually born susceptible, unless vertical transmission has occurred. In utero infection can occur, but most frequently in utero transmission will lead to abortion or stillborn calves (Hinton, 1974). Upon exposure, there is a very short latent period (12-48 hours). For practical purposes, this latent period can often be disregarded because it is so short. The animal will then begin to excrete bacteria - mainly in faeces. At this point, the host is considered infectious. The infectious period varies tremendously between individuals, both with regard to duration and the amounts of bacteria being shed. Not all animals are clinically affected during the infectious period, and those that are may not remain ill for the full duration of the infectious period. Furthermore, antibiotic treatment has little relevant effect on control. Some treated calves stop shedding bacteria, but continue to show clinical signs. Other treated calves stop exhibiting clinical signs, but still excrete the bacteria - and there are even suggestions that in some cases, a persistent carrier stage may develop upon treatment with an antibiotic. In other words, it is difficult to provide a prognosis for the course of infection; regarding both clinical signs, and for subclinical infections that usually go unnoticed in infected herds.

There are suggestions in the literature that *S.* Dublin may lead to a prolonged infection stage in a small proportion of animals (the 'carriers' or 'persistent carriers' that excrete bacteria either continuously or intermittently). Some cattle become latently infected and do not shed bacteria to such an extent that it is detectable. However, the bacteria may potentially become reactivated during stressful events in the animal's life cycle, and they can begin to excrete higher amounts of bacteria for shorter or longer durations. Hence, such carriers may contribute importantly to the epidemiology of *S.* Dublin in infected herds (House et al., 1993; Nielsen et al., 2012a; Nielsen et al., 2004a; Richardson, 1973). Unfortunately, they are difficult to detect and differentiate from transiently infected (i.e. cattle that become infected and then clear the infection after a few days or weeks) and non-infected cattle (Lomborg et al., 2007; Nielsen, 2013b). It is important to note that cattle that have been infected once with *S.* Dublin can recover and lose their immunity after a variable length of time. They can therefore become reinfected and excrete bacteria again later in life (Steinbach et al., 1996). Fig. 11.3.1 illustrates the infection stages of *S.* Dublin that are most commonly described in the literature.

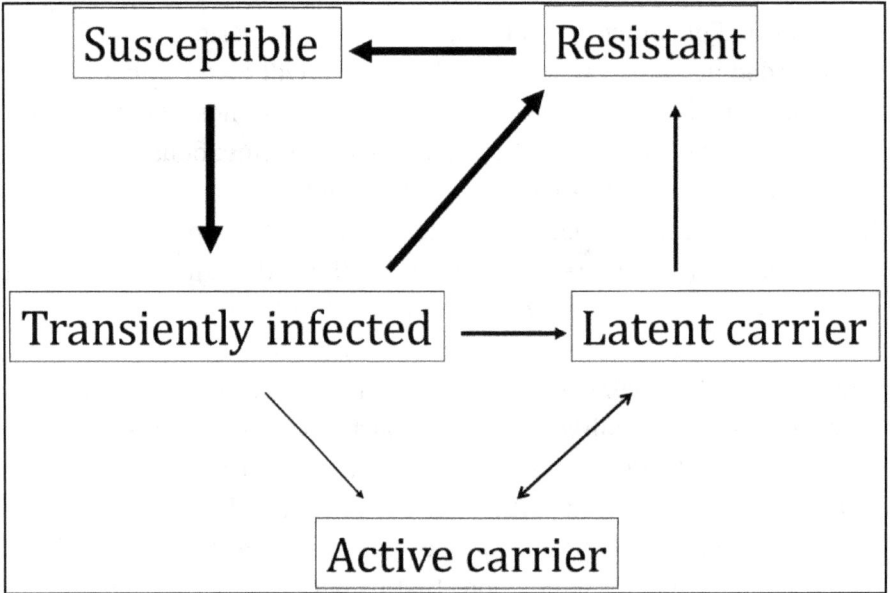

Figure 11.3.1. Overview of *S.* Dublin infection stages commonly described in the literature. The infectious stages where animals are excreting bacteria are referred to as transiently infected and active carriers. The latent carriers are infected, but do not excrete bacteria unless they become reactivated, and then they typically shed low concentrations of bacteria for a limited time period. Clinical signs may be present in the transiently infected stage to varying degrees. Production losses (e.g. reduced milk production and growth retardation) may be present in all stages of infection including animals that have recently recovered from infection (resistant).

However, terminology in literature is confusing, and there is controversy regarding the existence and importance of the different infection stages. An active carrier (or super-shedder) stage might be relevant for *S.* Dublin. Active carriers may continue to shed similar amounts of bacteria as transiently infected animals for an extended period of time (such as months). However, it appears from the limited evidence in literature that this only rarely occurs. It is therefore more likely that the latent stage, with no or rare reactivation of faecal excretion of bacteria, is the most common persistent *S.* Dublin infection, and such carriers therefore excrete markedly lower concentrations of bacteria than transiently infected animals (Sojka et al., 1974). This fits well with the fairly low probability of excretion found in cattle above 7 months old in a longitudinal study of endemically infected Danish dairy herds (Nielsen, 2013b). This suggests that the main focus in control of *S.* Dublin should be aimed at preventing spread of infection to and between young calves.

11.3.4. Transmission

Transmission can occur via uptake of *S.* Dublin bacteria excreted in faecal matter, in milk or - in rare cases - in utero. Infection via conjunctiva, airways and the teat canal is also possible, but is more of a curiosity than of practical importance for the epidemiology of the infection in cattle herds. Due to the long survival times and the potential to multiply outside the host, the environment is an important reservoir of infection, and plays an important role for indirect transmission between animals and farms (Hardman et al., 1991; Nielsen et al., 2007). Susceptibility is age-related, with calves being more susceptible to infection than older animals. Yet it is possible for any age group to be infected, and it is therefore necessary to consider potential transmission routes in all barn sections and all age groups.

The infectious dose of *S.* Dublin is strain-dependent (Wallis et al., 1995). Usually, oral uptake of more than 10^6 colony forming units (CFU) leads to clinical signs and/or shedding of bacteria in calves less than 6 months old. Pre-weaned calves are highly susceptible (Nazer and Osborne, 1977; Segall and Lindberg, 1991). In general, the higher the infection dose, the more consistently shedding and clinical signs can be reproduced experimentally. The environmental conditions and shedding pattern of infectious animals may be quite different under experimental settings from those in an ordinary farming setting. Therefore, susceptible hosts may be intermittently exposed to smaller doses of bacteria, leading to infections with fewer and milder clinical signs, and different patterns of excretion than those observed in experimental research (Wray and Sojka, 1981). In older cattle, experimentally administered oral doses of 10^{10}-10^{11} CFU have been found to lead to variable responses ranging from no clinical signs to severe illness with dysentery, pyrexia and abortions in pregnant heifers (Hall and Jones, 1979). Naturally infected cows aborting under field conditions often have few or no clinical signs other than an easily overlooked transient fever, but they may also be shedding bacteria in faeces around the time of abortion (Hinton, 1974; Richardson and Watson, 1971).

The most obvious way to break the transmission route for *S.* Dublin is therefore to limit contact between different age groups, as well as to avoid exposure of calves to faecal contamination from other animals in the herd, including calves and older cattle in the barn. Calves should be born in a clean environment (preferably a single calving pen so that it is only in contact with its own dam) and later moved into a clean calf pen or hut. Newborn calves should also be fed a sufficient amount of high quality colostrum within 6 hours to reduce their susceptibility to gastrointestinal pathogens. To allow the most natural behavioural development, it is necessary to allow contact with another calf of a similar age (but this should be limited to one other calf to prevent further spread of infectious agents). Should one animal become infectious, the bacteria have more opportunity to spread within the barn if a greater number of susceptible hosts are kept together. It is worth mentioning that aggressive cleaning procedures such as high-pressure washing should not be used in barn areas with animals present, as it may lead to spread of *S.* Dublin and other infectious agents through aerosols. This type of cleaning is effective to clean empty barns, pens and huts, but must be followed by drying out and disinfection in order to have the desired effect. Furthermore, protective clothing and facemasks must be worn during high-pressure washing. Otherwise, people are also at risk of becoming infected.

11.3.5. Diagnosis

Perfect diagnostic tests for *S.* Dublin do not exist - at animal level, or at herd level. The diagnosis of *S.* Dublin at animal level is challenged by the complexity of the pathogenesis - with several infection stages, and the varying bacterial excretion patterns and antibody levels produced by individual infected animals. The diagnostic methods available (as of 2013) for use in practice are reviewed by Nielsen (2013a). When using diagnostic procedures as part of the control and prevention of *S*. Dublin, one needs to accept use of 'probability diagnoses'. It is important to think about the target condition that the diagnostic test should detect, e.g. exposed, infected, infectious or diseased animals. The purpose of testing to see whether animals have been exposed to *S*. Dublin is very different from testing for infectiousness. If the purpose is to detect infectious animals (so that these can be culled or isolated from the rest of the herd) we may choose to use repeated faecal culture. Unfortunately, faecal culture has poor Se, i.e. not generally higher than 50%, and often much lower than that due to intermittent shedding in low concentrations (Nielsen et al., 2004b). We are therefore likely to overlook some infectious animals if we rely too heavily on faecal culture. Furthermore, collecting the faecal material is time-consuming and the laboratory test is expensive compared to antibody-detecting ELISAs, for example. On the other hand, presence of antibodies in serum or milk does not indicate whether or not the animal is infectious, but merely shows that the animal has been exposed to *S*. Dublin bacteria at some time in the past. It has been suggested that repeated antibody measurements taken twice over a period of 60 days can be used to detect persistently infected carriers (Spier et al., 1990). However, recent studies suggest that there is low probability of excretion in animals with persistently high antibody titres in endemically infected herds. Hence, testing-and-culling of potential persistent carriers is not recommended as the only or main diagnostic test-strategy in a successful control programme (Nielsen, 2013b).

In the Danish *S*. Dublin control and eradication programmes, a frequently used and recommended approach is to screen dairy herds using a BTM ELISA, and non-dairy herds using blood samples from the herd, with the number of blood samples to be taken determined by the herd size. Herd testing methods and the associated herd level Se and Sp are reviewed by Nielsen (2013c). It is recommended to initiate an action plan with test-positive herds, and to perform regular ELISA testing (e.g. every 3-6 months) on the ten youngest calves above 3 months old, in order to evaluate whether the plan is still working. Calves between 3-6 months old generally do not have *S*. Dublin antibodies unless they have been exposed to the bacteria. Hence, if all ten calves have an antibody level of close to zero, this is a strong indication that transmission of bacteria has been prevented in the young calves. Once it has been established that effective practices to prevent spread of bacteria are in place, it may be worth initiating repeated antibody measurements of older cattle to identify adult heifers or cows that remain persistently high, while the antibody levels in the rest of the herd decrease. These individuals present a significantly higher probability of excreting bacteria than others in their herd, and may therefore be recommended for culling (Nielsen, 2013b). However, it is not possible to distinguish these individuals from transiently infected animals when transmission in the herd is ongoing.

11.3.6. Epidemiology

Very few countries have national surveillance programmes, nor perform regular surveys to estimate the national herd-level prevalence of *S.* Dublin in their cattle populations. Therefore, there are few estimates with which to compare the Danish prevalence. Fig. 11.3.2 shows the development in the national apparent prevalence (AP), and estimated true prevalence (TP) of *S.* Dublin in Danish dairy herds between 2002 (when sampling of all herds was initiated and the AP was close to 25%) and July 2014 (when the AP was 6.1% and the estimated TP was 4.4%). The interpretation is that in July 2014, 6.1% of the dairy herds had serological reactions in the BTM above the limits dictated in the Danish herd classification programme. However, only 4.4% of the dairy herds were actually infected. The case definition of herd infection was that if all animals were sampled individually by milk or blood samples within the herd, at least one animal would test positive in faecal culture, or more than 5% of the individual animals would test positive by ELISA (Warnick et al., 2006). The main reason for the discrepancy between AP and TP is because of the time delay between the clearance of *Salmonella* bacteria from the herd, and the point at which the antibody levels in individual cows have reduced sufficiently for the herd to be classified as test-negative in the herd classification programme. Furthermore, there are likely some herds that are infected with other serotypes than *S.* Dublin, but they may react in the *S.* Dublin-ELISA due to cross-reaction between common O-antigens on the bacterial cell surfaces (Konrad et al., 1994).

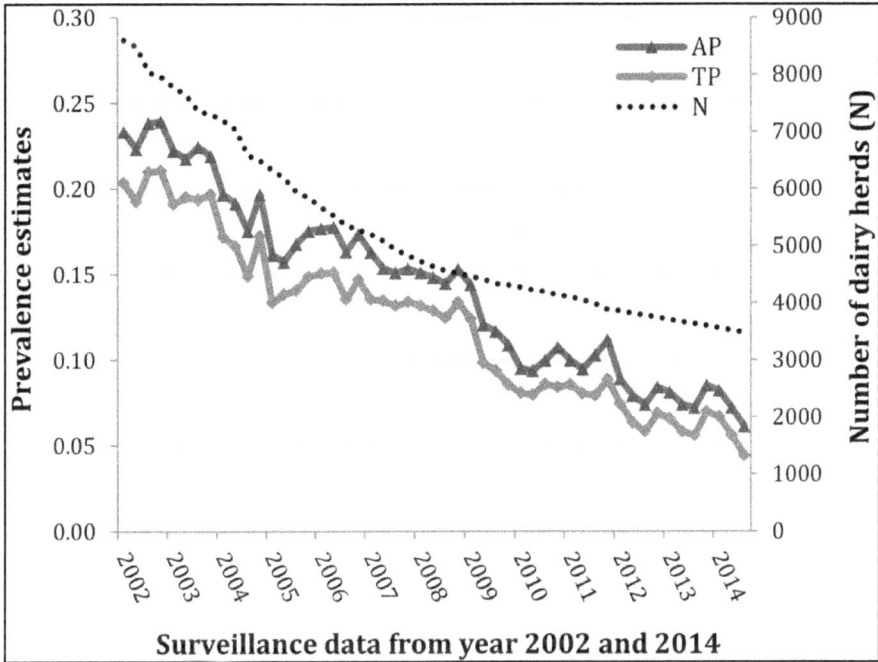

Figure 11.3.2. The apparent prevalence (AP), estimated true prevalence (TP) and number of dairy herds (N) shown quarterly between January 2002 and July 2014 according to the Danish surveillance programme for *S.* Dublin. The TP was calculated based on the AP and known herd-level Se and Sp of the test-procedures used in the programme for herd classification.

Within infected herds the prevalence can vary considerably. *S.* Dublin is a very dynamic infection, spreading rapidly and generating herd immunity, which consequently reduces the within-herd prevalence until a new wave of infection occurs. As a result, approximately annual waves of infection are common under Danish farming conditions (Nielsen, 2013d; Nielsen et al., 2012a). Therefore the seroprevalence periodically reaches more than 80%, whereas the prevalence of faecal culture positive animals rarely exceeds 25%. However, this may also be due to the low diagnostic Se of faecal culture to detect infected animals. Generally, younger cattle excrete *S.* Dublin more frequently and in higher concentrations than adult cattle within infected herds.

The duration of infection in infected herds varies with herd size, management and hygiene levels in the farm. The effect of herd size can be attributed to more animals being present to be infected and spread the infection, and therefore the larger the herd is, the lower the probability that the infection will die out by chance. Management affects the hygiene level and other biosecurity parameters such as direct contact between animals. The animals' susceptibility may be also affected by housing, handling and feeding strategies in the farm. Good barn environment hygiene and limited contact between animals have been shown to be very important elements of successful control (Nielsen et al., 2012a; Nielsen et al., 2012b).

11.3.7. Effects of S. Dublin infection

S. Dublin increases mortality and morbidity in affected herds (causing clinical signs such as diarrhoea, pneumonia, fever, septic arthritis, abortions, and weight loss). Moreover, the infection has recently been shown to affect milk production in infected dairy herds to a greater extent than was previously expected. Since it is now possible to evaluate the effects against long-term surveillance data, it has become clear that S. Dublin has a marked effect on milk production; both during outbreaks and in endemically infected herds (Nielsen et al., 2013). In lactating cows, it was found to be associated with fairly large milk yield losses (i.e. up to 3 energy-corrected kg of milk (ECM) per day in third parity cows, for an extended period of months or years after the introduction of the infection to the herd).

In general, disease and mortality patterns follow epidemic waves in infected herds. However, an interesting pattern has been shown for acute infections and abortions in adult cattle after the first 2 years of herd infection. Repeated infection of YS in herds with poor control of the infection leads to a high proportion of resistant adult cattle, which in turn leads to a reduction in the number of acute infections in adults, and thus relatively fewer associated abortions (Nielsen et al., 2012a). This phenomenon of resistance among adult cattle explains why some farmers do not perceive the presence of S. Dublin in their herd as a problem, despite milk production being potentially lower due to the continued presence of the infection. However, estimated gross margin losses in endemically infected herds proportioned for 200 cows were between EUR 1,400 and 34,600 per year, depending on the extent of infection spread within the herd, which again is related to management and hygiene (Nielsen et al., 2013).

If the economic effects of *S.* Dublin infection are summarised nationally at a prevalence of 4.4% in dairy herds, this leads to estimated gross margin losses of at least EUR 2.3 million per year for the Danish cattle sector of approximately 550,000 dairy cows. In years with high milk prices, the losses are even larger. Hence, the effect on production alone justifies the strategy to eradicate the infection from the cattle population. In addition, the reduction of animal welfare associated with disease occurrence, as well as production losses in the slaughter calf production sector, and the zoonotic risk to consumers should be considered when evaluating the benefits of eradicating *S.* Dublin from the dairy cattle sector.

11.3.8. The Danish surveillance and control programme for *S.* Dublin

The effects of the infection on animal health and welfare, production economics and food safety demonstrated the need to control *S.* Dublin in Denmark. The motivation for choosing a mandatory programme inclusive of all cattle herds was mainly politically led, but was also scientifically meaningful because of the high risk of transmission between cattle farms. If not all herds were classified in the programme, there would be a higher risk of reinfection from non-enrolled, infected herds. The primary reasons for the mandatory programme provided were that: a) *S.* Dublin is an important zoonosis, and although it is rarely seen in humans, it is associated with high case-fatality, b) *S.* Dublin was associated with morbidity and mortality in infected herds and about 25% of the dairy herds were estimated to be infected in the late 1990s, c) the other primary sectors (i.e. eggs, poultry and pigs) had successful salmonella control programmes in place, and there was a national policy to reduce the incidence of human salmonellosis, so the political pressure on the cattle sector to act was increasing, and d) it was no longer considered sufficient to rely on passive surveillance (i.e. reporting of clinical cases or clinical suspicions) to detect infected herds and control the spread from only these herds.

Hence, a mandatory national surveillance programme covering all Danish cattle herds was initiated in October 2002. From the very beginning, the steering committee of the programme lead by the Danish Veterinary and Food Administration, decided that herd classification should be publicly available via the official Central Husbandry Register so that farmers could protect their herd when purchasing replacement stock. Furthermore, a rule was included in the legislation that a test-negative ('Level 1') farm would be locked in a test-positive ('Level 2') surveillance classification for at least 3 months when purchasing cattle from a test-positive farm, in order to prevent further spread of infection in the event that the purchasing herd became infected. Initially, this was a very unpopular arrangement, as it made the farmers feel exposed and many were afraid of receiving negative attention from the public or other farmers. However, it had a dramatic effect on the trading behaviour. The proportion of farmers with test-negative herds purchasing cattle from test-positive herds dropped from around 40% to below 5% within the first 6 months after programme initiation, and this restrictive purchase pattern continued. It is most likely that this was the main reason for the prevalence reductions observed during the first years of the Danish *S.* Dublin surveillance programme. After about 1 year, farmers became familiar with the herd classification programme, and started using it more deliberately for control purposes.

Research projects showed that aside from external biosecurity (restricting trade of live animals), the most important control measures in stopping infection spread within infected herds included hygiene and management aimed at reducing contact; both between infected and non-infected animals, and susceptible animals and the environment. It also became evident that the available diagnostic tests were most suitable in test-strategies aimed at assessing progress in the control action plan rather than actual test-and-cull strategies. The main incentive for farmers was to be classified 'Level 1' which would open up new trading opportunities, but some farmers also reacted simply because it was undesirable to be classified as 'Level 2'. Finally, some farmers began controlling the infection, because they became aware that the clinical problems in their herd were associated with *S.* Dublin. During the programme, extensive communication was provided to farmers and their local advisors through courses, articles in farmer magazines, at farmers' conferences, by direct letters to specific types of farms, at information meetings and through different types of field and research project. A homepage with a continual update of knowledge and information sources to assist farmers and local advisors was created at: www.salmonella.dk. Throughout the programme, all the important stakeholders including farmers' organisations, the veterinary authorities, the public health authorities, laboratories, the veterinary association and universities were involved in working groups, an advisory board and the steering committee. At the beginning of the programme, the resources used for the surveillance programme mainly came from CO_2 funds that were collected from farmers as production fees and directed back to the farming industry by the government. Most other resources were allocated through the farmers' own organisations (e.g. Cattle and Milk Levy Funds and other types of project funding).

The surveillance programme was successful in markedly reducing the prevalence during the first couple of years. However in 2006, the 'Level 2' classification lock-in period following purchase or contact to test-positive herds was reduced from 3 months to 3 weeks due to farmer complaints that the regulations made it too difficult to run a business, especially for breeding herds. From 2005 to 2007 the AP remained stable at around 15-18%, and the cattle sector, in collaboration with the Danish Veterinary and Food Administration, looked for alternative methods to further reduce the prevalence. A research project revealed that reduction in the duration of infection was critical to reduce the prevalence in infected herds further (Jordan et al., 2008). Consequently, in 2007 the decision was made to change the programme from a surveillance to an eradication programme, with the aim to eradicate *S. Dublin* from the Danish cattle population by end of 2014. Three phases were planned:

Phase 1: 2007-2009 Voluntary control efforts supported by research and field projects.

Phase 2: 2010-2012 Increase motivation to eliminate the infection from infected herds by implementing further restrictions and consequences in the legislation.

Phase 3: 2013-2014 Restrictive handling of infected herds by the regional veterinary offices.

To kick-start the voluntary control efforts in Phase 1, and to provide evidence of effective approaches to control *S.* Dublin in infected herds, a pilot study was initiated in 2007 in South Jutland. The pilot study was successful, so in 2008 the decision was made to use the same approach to eradicate *S.* Dublin in the rest of the country (see below). Throughout the control and eradication programmes, the surveillance programme continued to provide straightforward follow-up on the effect of different initiatives, new ministerial orders in 2002, 2006, 2010, 2012, 2013, and 2014, and changing conditions, e.g. in the structural changes of the cattle population.

11.3.9. A pilot study and new control initiatives

A pilot study was initiated in 2007 in the South Jutland region in an attempt to improve within-herd control efforts using a stable-school approach. It was hoped that this would motivate farmers to implement the right management procedures in their farms (Vaarst et al., 2007). A total of 212 farmers with 'Level 2' herds were invited to participate, and 105 of them decided to join a network of farmers who visited other farms in the group ('stable-schools') to learn from and support each other. Evaluations of the project indicated that participating farmers appreciated the approach, and the effect on surveillance data from participating farms compared to non-participating farms was so promising that the approach was implemented in the rest of the Jutland peninsula, because Jutland had the highest prevalence of *S.* Dublin. Interestingly, as the prevalence of test-positive herds plummeted, the farmer-driven pressure on their own organisation for further initiatives to limit the spread from the infected herds to the test-negative herds increased throughout the country.

In 2010 it was decided that the network group approach had outlived its usefulness. Most of the farmers that were motivated by this approach had already participated in network groups, and with the national prevalence now hovering around 10%, new initiatives were required to reduce the prevalence even further. Phase 2 of the eradication programme began by changing the legislation to considerably restrict movement of cattle out of test-positive herds. Essentially, only movements directly to slaughter or export were allowed. One exception was that it became possible to sell young calves to slaughter calf producers who had signed contracts accepting calves from *S.* Dublin test-positive dairy herds. In addition, a project aiming to encourage slaughter calf producers to prevent introduction of *S.* Dublin to their herds was initiated. In practice, this was achieved by the slaughter calf producers demanding proof of antibody negative calves from the delivering herds. Furthermore, they increased their focus on avoiding purchase of ill-thriven calves. This produced an indirect pressure on 'Level 2' dairy farmers, but also affected them directly as the market price of calves sold from 'Level 2' herds dropped to about half the price of calves from 'Level 1'.

However, phase 2 of the eradication programme did not have the desired effect, and by end of 2012 it was clear that stricter legislation was required to reduce the prevalence even further than the 8.3% test-positive dairy herds. Furthermore, the aim of the programme was adjusted to *S.* Dublin being eradicated from the Danish cattle population by end of 2016. A new legislative order was put in place in July 2013. The new initiatives included regionalisation of Denmark into a low-prevalence region (the islands) and a high-prevalence region (the peninsula of Jutland). Test-positive herds in the low-prevalence region were put under official veterinary supervision, and it was mandatory for test-positive herds in the high-prevalence region to make a targeted action plan, followed by sampling of at least ten young calves every 3 months to evaluate the effect of the action plan. The herd classification scheme dictated by the legislative order from July 2013 is summarised in Table 11.3.1. A map of the distribution of test-positive herds in Denmark on 5 May 2010 and on 30 July 2014 is shown in Fig. 11.3.3.

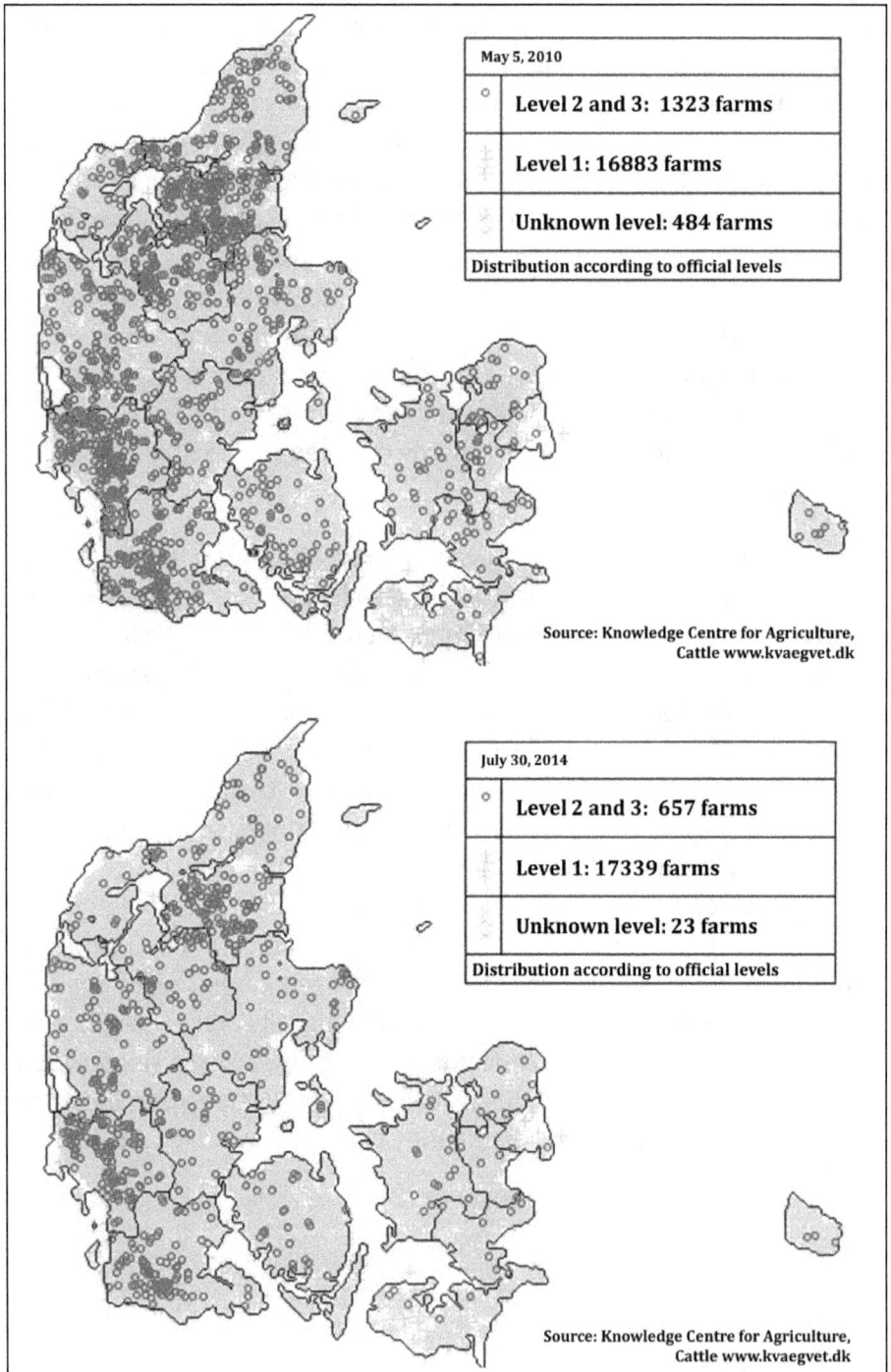

May 5, 2010

○	**Level 2 and 3: 1323 farms**
	Level 1: 16883 farms
	Unknown level: 484 farms

Distribution according to official levels

Source: Knowledge Centre for Agriculture,
Cattle www.kvaegvet.dk

July 30, 2014

○	**Level 2 and 3: 657 farms**
	Level 1: 17339 farms
	Unknown level: 23 farms

Distribution according to official levels

Source: Knowledge Centre for Agriculture,
Cattle www.kvaegvet.dk

Figure 11.3.3. Distribution of test-positive cattle herds in Denmark in 2010 (top) and 2014 (bottom) (source: Knowledge Centre for Agriculture, Cattle, www.kvaegvet.dk, accessed 30 July 2014).

Table 11.3.1. An overview of the herd classification scheme in the Danish *S.* Dublin surveillance programme for cattle herds according the legislative order issued in July 2013 (Anonymous, 2013).

Surveillance level	Official interpretation	Criteria	Consequences dictated by legislation
Level 1	Most likely free from *S.* Dublin infection	*Dairy herds:* Average optical density corrected (ODC)%<25 in the last four BTM samples and that had not increased >20 ODC% in the last sample compared to the average of the previous three samples *For non-dairy herds:* The last (up to) eight blood samples from the herd <50 ODC% (the sample size depends on the herd size)	Level 1 herds in the low prevalence region ('the Islands') cannot purchase cattle from the high-prevalence region (the peninsula, Jutland). Level 1 herds in the high-prevalence region cannot sell/move cattle to the low-prevalence region unless directly to a slaughter calf producer who only produces cattle for slaughter.
Level 2	Possibly infected based high antibody levels, risky contacts or unknown status due to too few samples	*For dairy herds:* BTM values above cut-off defined for Level 1 *For non-dairy herds:* At least one of the last up to eight blood samples from the herd ≥50 ODC% *For all herd types*: Purchase or other types of recorded contact to herds not classified as Level 1 Bacteriological culture positive but no signs of salmonellosis	Level 2 herds in the low-prevalence region put under official veterinary supervision (closed herd – can only deliver to slaughter) Level 2 herds in high-prevalence region must make an action plan for *S.* Dublin with follow-up sampling to evaluate the effect of the plan. Cannot move animals to other farms (with few exceptions).
Level 3	Confirmed clinical salmonellosis	Clinical signs of salmonellosis + *S.* Dublin confirmed by bacteriological culture	Herd put under official veterinary supervision by veterinary authorities, can only send animals to slaughter for special hygienic slaughter lines.

11.4. Paratuberculosis

11.4.1. Introduction

Paratuberculosis is a chronic infection caused by *Mycobacterium avium* subsp. *paratuberculosis* (MAP). The infection has been recognised for over 100 years, and methods of controlling the infection have been pursued for an equally long time. The primary effects of infection are chronic intermittent diarrhoea ultimately leading to death, reduced milk yield and slaughter weight, and there is also a possible risk of MAP being zoonotic (Behr and Kapur, 2008; Kudahl et al., 2009; Nielsen et al., 2009; Raizman et al., 2007). Consequently, animal health and welfare, farming profitability and food safety might all be affected by MAP infections, and control of MAP could address one or more of these effects.

Challenges in the control and eradication include: a) the chronic nature of the disease, where not all infected animals become diseased during their lifetime; b) the lack of accurate tests to detect MAP infections in early stages of infection; c) poor understanding and use of the diagnostic tests in a fit-for-purpose framework; d) long survival of MAP in the environment; and e) lack of motivated farmers due to variable effects on farming profitability, and difficulties in determining whether MAP impacts food safety. Several aspects including the pathogen and its effect on the host are of importance, and along with transmission and epidemiology, will be described briefly before a discussion of elements of the Danish MAP programme.

11.4.2. *Mycobacterium avium* subsp. *paratuberculosis* (MAP)

MAP are slow-growing, acid-fast bacteria with visible growth often only occurring after 8-12 weeks of incubation on solid media (Hirsh and Biberstein, 2004). Historically, MAP were considered to be non-spore forming, but recent data suggest that they may enter a spore-like dormant stage, where they are extremely resistant to external factors such as heat (Lamont et al., 2012). This may also explain their ability to survive for a long time within the host (Coussens et al., 2009), and for years in the environment and water (Whittington et al., 2004; 2005). Although limited information is available on the topic, disinfectants are not thought to be effective against MAP. However, removal of faecal matter should be effective in eliminating the primary source of infection.

Animal-derived MAP can be discriminated from other mycobacteria by the repetitive DNA sequence IS900, which is considered to be specific to MAP (Collins et al., 1989). Strain types of apparently varying pathogenicity have been identified, but identification of differences in virulence for specific strain types is still an area in its infancy (Stevenson, 2009).

11.4.3. Pathogenesis

Uptake of MAP is usually via the faecal-oral route. MAP can be ingested from faeces or contaminated feed, milk, water and environment; or transferred in utero (Sweeney, 2011; Sweeney et al., 1992; Whittington and Windsor, 2009). Once MAP has been ingested, it will usually enter via the tonsils or via the M-cells in the ileal Peyer patches (Momotani et al., 1988; Payne and Rankin, 1961). The bacteria are ingested by macrophages, in which they persist and replicate, eventually forming granulomas. The killing of MAP in the macrophage may be achieved through phagosome acidification with subsequent phagosome-lysosome fusion and MAP destruction. However, MAP may be able to survive the attack by the macrophage, proceed to kill the macrophage and spread to neighbouring cells. Granuloma formation is then initiated. The form and extent of the granulomatous response depend upon the immune response. The initial immune response is likely to be an effective pro-inflammatory response dominated by Th1-cells. One commonly recorded marker of this response is interferon-γ (IFN-γ). IFN-γ is usually associated with limited focal lesions, whereas multifocal to diffuse forms are associated with Th2-responses and the occurrence of IgG1 (Immunoglobulin G) antibodies (Vazquez et al., 2013). While the pro-inflammatory response is considered to be 'effective' in killing MAP, it is not known whether eradication of the pathogen from the animal (i.e. a 'cure') is indeed possible. However, occurrence of IgG1 antibodies is an indicator that control of the infection has been lost (Stabel, 2006), and that high levels of excretion of MAP, reduced body mass and reduced milk yield are likely to follow (Kudahl and Nielsen, 2009b; Nielsen, 2008; Nielsen et al., 2009). Eventually, the animal will develop chronic diarrhoea and die from the infection. The mechanisms involved in control or progression of MAP infections are unknown, but not all infected animals develop clinical disease: either because they can control the infection, or because the incubation period can vary significantly and be longer than the lifetime of many cattle.

11.4.4. Transmission

Horizontal transmission of MAP can be direct and indirect: transmission can occur via uptake of MAP excreted in faecal matter and in milk; but vertical transmission can also occur in utero. Due to the potentially long survival periods, the environment can act as a MAP reservoir. There is a distinct age-related susceptibility, with calves being more susceptible to infection than older animals (Taylor, 1953). Infection of adult cattle is still considered possible (Larsen et al., 1975; Mitchell et al., 2012), but the proportion of infected animals is lower and the progression of infection slower. The extent of bacterial excretion varies with infection stage. Newly infected animals may excrete MAP in early calfhood, after which this excretion usually ceases (van Roermund et al., 2007). However, the infection dose is speculated to have a huge impact on the course of the infection, and more persistent shedding has been observed in experiments where the animals have been infected with high doses of MAP (Lepper et al., 1989). The combination of infection dose, number of exposures and age appears to affect the duration of this early excretion period as well as the course of infection (Mitchell et al., 2012). However, the relation between dose and response in the pathogenesis is still poorly understood. To summarise in simple terms, calves should not be exposed to faeces and milk of infectious cows, but it should be acknowledged that adults may also be infected if subjected to large quantities of MAP. In utero transmission is also possible, and calves born infected or those infected in calfhood may transmit MAP to their herd-mates.

11.4.5. Diagnosis

Diagnosis of MAP infections is hampered by the chronic nature of the infection. Highly accurate tests do not exist because of the protracted pathogenesis. Furthermore, the uncertainty over whether an infection can be cured, or whether it will eventually lead to disease if the animal lives long enough, also adds to the diagnostic difficulties. It is therefore essential to be clear on the purpose of testing in relation to control of the infection in order to establish a reasonable MAP diagnosis. A recent review outlines the use of diagnostic tests for different purposes (Nielsen, 2014a). Briefly, BTM tests are not deemed to be effective, because they are too insensitive and non-specific to be of diagnostic value. Establishing whether a herd is infected can be the first step in a control scheme. For this purpose, strategic sampling from the environment or from subsets of cows may provide a crude diagnosis, particularly if the prevalence is high (Lombard et al., 2013). The samples can be subject to bacteriological analyses using culture or PCR, or detection of antibodies. The latter may result in non-specific reactions. The herd Se is highly dependent on the within-herd prevalence and the number of samples collected. At a low prevalence, even hundreds of samples may be insufficient to detect infected herds (Tavornpanich et al., 2012).

If a herd is deemed to be infected, bacteriological or immunological tests can be used at animal level. Multiple tests and test-strategies are available, and at the time of writing no single test-strategy is considered superior to the others. However, both bacteriological and immunological tests may be result in false-positive reactions for the individual, and it is therefore important to be aware of this possibility when communicating test-positive reactions. In general, the decisions made based on test-results should be clearly outlined in a test-and-management strategy. Without this, testing should not be performed.

11.4.6. Epidemiology

MAP infections appear to be widespread globally, including most of the cattle populations where MAP-targeted prevalence studies have been carried out. However, many MAP prevalence studies do not provide interpretable prevalence estimates, and useful data are scarce (Nielsen and Toft, 2009). The primary reasons are poor reporting, poorly designed studies, lack of consistency in target conditions across studies, challenges in establishing a diagnosis, and inaccurate and imprecise diagnostic tests. One example of the challenges in prevalence estimation and interpreting reported prevalences is the apparent 'increase' in prevalences of infected herds. A study conducted in the USA in 1996 revealed a herd-level prevalence of 22%, where an infected herd was supposedly defined as herds with ≥10% infected animals (NAHMS, 1997), but a NAHMS study with sampling in 2007 revealed a 'true herd-level prevalence' of 91% (Lombard et al., 2013). However, the two estimates are not really comparable. Differences in study design, diagnostic tests and target conditions are the likely primary reasons for the differences in the reported prevalences, although a real increase in the herd-level prevalence is also a likely contributor to the differences. Minor differences in definitions, test interpretation, study designs etc. can develop into major differences when data are interpreted on regional or national level. For example, the prevalence estimates based on data from the Danish control programme on paratuberculosis could be quite different depending on choices of apparently 'minor' details made in the estimation process as illustrated in Fig. 11.4.1. In particular, the estimation of between-herd prevalences would be affected by the low within-herd prevalences. In this example, between-herd prevalence estimates ranged from between 49% to 86% by simply making small changes in interpretation of the data. However, in most countries with a significant dairy cattle production, it appears that between-herd infection prevalences are generally above 50% and within-herd prevalences are quite variable (Nielsen and Toft, 2009). These prevalences are likely to be influenced by the herd demographics, particularly herd size and introduction of animals from other herds (Nielsen and Toft, 2011).

11.4.7. Effects of MAP infection

Currently, we do not know if all MAP infections would result in every possible adverse effect, should the animal live for long enough. We might be required to address the various effects differently, depending on their nature (e.g. impact on production traits or zoonotic potential). At animal level, the adverse effects might include:

- Reduced milk yield;
- Reduced body condition eventually resulting in emaciation and death;
- Intermittent or chronic diarrhoea.

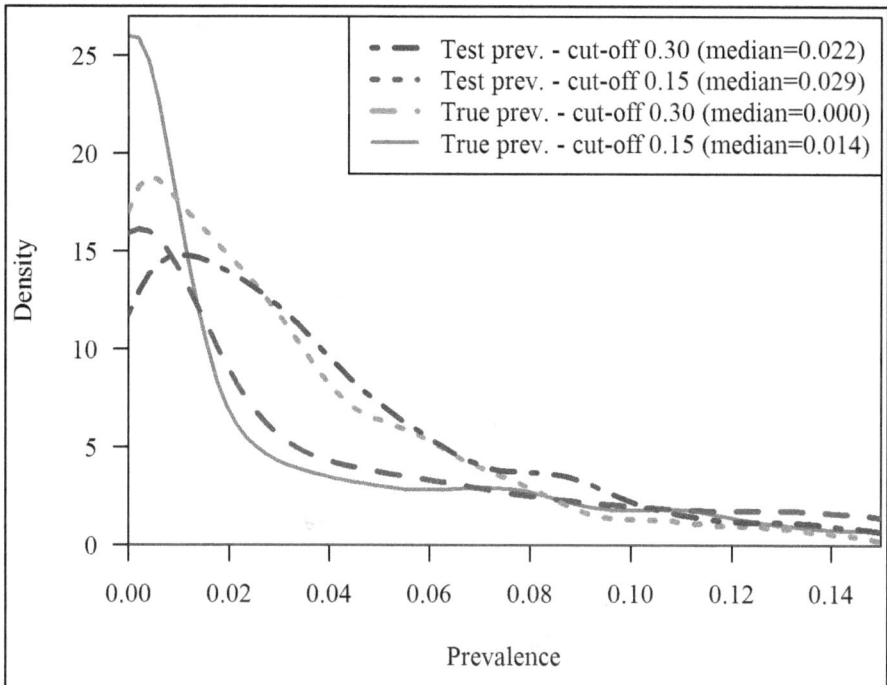

Figure 11.4.1. Within-herd prevalence distribution among 1,008 Danish dairy cattle herds in the Danish control programme as of March 2013, based on different ways to assess the prevalence: using the test-prevalence i.e. ELISA-positive at two different cut-offs in ID-Screen (ID-Vet, Grabels, France), 0.15, as recommended by the producer, and another arbitrary value (0.30). At both cut-offs, the TP was then estimated using Sp and age-specific Se estimates as reported in Nielsen et al. (2013). Despite the fact that the underlying data were the same, relatively different distributions were achieved, illustrating that the choices greatly impact the estimates. The resulting between-herd prevalences would have been 0.86 and 0.79 based on test-prevalences at cut-offs 0.15 and 0.30, respectively, whereas the between-herd prevalences would be 0.59 and 0.49 based on the TP at cut-offs 0.15 and 0.30, respectively.

Excretion of MAP in infectious doses may not be considered an adverse effect to the excreting cow, but is a risk to her herd-mates and therefore primarily something of interest at herd level. Similarly, the adverse effect of 'non-progressed infection' and 'MAP excretion' may primarily be considered factors of interest in relation to the herd, whereas reduced milk yield, body condition, emaciation and diarrhoea are more related to the individual. Ultimately, they may all contribute to a reduction in profitability for the farmer. At farm level, the adverse effects therefore include:

- Reduced animal welfare (e.g. emaciated cows and cows with diarrhoea);
- Increased internal transmission (retaining MAP in the herd);
- Increased external transmission (reducing the value of livestock for sale);
- Reduced milk production;
- Reduced slaughter value.

The summarised effects, costs and potential savings can be assessed in cost-benefit analyses and in models assessing the technical and economic effects following different management strategies (Kudahl et al., 2008). Summary measures at herd level (Richardson and More, 2009) or national level (Ott et al., 1999) may be used to determine if a herd, regional or national programme should be initiated.

<u>11.4.8. Control programmes</u>

Various MAP control schemes have been implemented in different countries over the past century. Many of the first were based on vaccination (Benedictus et al., 2000). It is generally acknowledged that control efforts should focus on reducing the between-herd spread of MAP by restricting movement of infected livestock, and within-herd transmission should be reduced by implementing measures to reduce the spread of MAP (Groenendaal et al., 2003). Consequently, more recent programmes place a great deal of focus on measures to reduce transmission via improved biosecurity, although the objectives of the different programmes vary extensively (Nielsen, 2009b). Limited success has been achieved regionally or nationally in these programmes, most likely due to the lack of consensus on the aim and purposes. Major challenges include proper implementation of the strategies described in scientific literature along with programme management. The ParaTB Forum was founded in Copenhagen in 2005 to assist programme managers in sharing experiences in existing and emerging programmes. The ParaTB Forum meetings have since taken place in Shanghai (2006),

Minneapolis (2009), Sydney (2012) and Parma (2014) with the proceedings from these meetings detailing the efforts available from www.paratuberculosis.info

11.4.9. Danish voluntary MAP control programme

The Danish control programme on paratuberculosis began in 2006 as a voluntary programme. The motivation and primary reasons for a voluntary approach was to engage individual farmers who had experienced production losses, or were concerned with potential future implications for loss and animal health, and therefore wished to control MAP (Nielsen, 2011). The Danish cattle industry also wished to gain experience in running such a programme, and the communication process played a major role. Stakeholders were identified and some included in an advisory board to provide input on central elements that should be communicated to farmers and advisors (Nielsen et al., 2007). Prior to the programme, a number of studies were carried out to address specific research questions (Nielsen, 2009a) and to engage farmers in understanding of the disease.

The aims of the programme were therefore twofold: a) to reduce the MAP infection prevalence in participating herds; and b) to provide farmers with tools to do so (Nielsen et al., 2007). The cattle industry thus provided the system and setup, while the individual farmers and their advisors established control efforts in practice. They were assisted in doing so through a common risk-based strategy recommended by the Danish Cattle Federation. This strategy included the following: a) quarterly testing of all lactating cows using an indirect ELISA for detection of MAP-specific antibodies in milk recording samples, with subsequent classification of cows into high ('red'), medium ('yellow') and low ('green') risk; b) disparate management of cows, based on their risk profile, at calving and at colostrum and milk feeding; and c) a recommendation not to purchase cows, or if necessary, only to purchase animals from tested, low-prevalence herds. Details on use of the diagnostics for risk-based management are available in different publications (Nielsen, 2007; 2009c). However, the risk-based approach may not necessarily be the most cost-effective in all dairy herds (Kudahl et al., 2008). The choice of strategy may rather depend on the hourly wages, practicalities of the herd etc. The reason for choosing the risk-based strategy as the primary recommended strategy was therefore more the result of the combination of the following elements: a) it should be cost-effective in the majority of situations; b) it should include regular testing to allow farmers to follow the development in prevalence; c) it should include as little management or additional work for the farmer as possible; and d) frequent testing would be a frequent reminder of the programme, so it would not be overlooked among all other daily routines.

The test-strategy thus played a central role in the initial programme design, despite the fact that control should be feasible without testing (Groenendaal et al., 2003). However, the availability of test information was deemed to be central to farmers' engagement, and consequently the risk-based approach was chosen. The test information was used for the purposes specified in Table 11.4.1.

Other tests can be used in a programme for different purposes (Nielsen, 2014a), but they were considered unnecessary in this particular programme. This decision could easily be challenged, but keeping the number of different tests to a minimum was pivotal to the implementation of test information and communication. This was particularly relevant for communication of the test-results, which were already complicated by the nature of the disease.

Education and communication were central parts of the establishment of the programme (Nielsen et al., 2007). This included establishment of an advisory board including programme managers, recording managers, laboratory managers, herd health advisors and a scientist. All were appointed based on their hands-on experience rather than their hierarchical status in the political or organisational society. They should, in other words, be influential on account of their skills, not their status. Furthermore, courses were organised for those requesting courses, and information was provided for those seeking information to self-educate (provided at a website http://www.paratuberkulose.dk). In addition, information was made available in varying degrees of detail in order to target those with a desire for detail, as well as those wishing only for summary information.

Table 11.4.1. Purposes, interpretation and actions associated with the use of diagnostic testing in the Danish control programme on paratuberculosis. The test-strategy includes four annual herd screenings using indirect ELISA for detection of MAP-specific antibodies in milk recording samples from individual cows.

Purpose	Interpretation	Action
Identify infectious animals	Occurrence of antibodies is an indicator that excretion of MAP is occurring or will occur in the near future. However, not all ELISA-positive animals have antibodies or excrete bacteria. Therefore, cows are separated into three risk groups: high risk ('red'), medium risk ('yellow') and low risk ('green')	Cull 'red' cows Special management of 'yellow' cows Do nothing about 'green' cows
Monitor efforts via prevalence	Early interpretation for: a) estimation of production loss; b) establishment of culling strategy: weak positive culled at low prevalence, whereas at a high prevalence MAP test-results could be combined with other information Later interpretation: decrease in prevalence among first parity cows a measure of success of biosecurity measures	Cull according to strategy Modify biosecurity if needed
Herd certification	Test-prevalences converted to infection prevalences and probability of low risk of being infected (according to Sergeant et al., 2008), combined with trading patterns used to establish 'certification levels'	Avoid purchase of livestock; or purchase low risk cattle only

The challenges in a voluntary programme are different to those in a mandatory programme. Establishment of success criteria are different, for example in a mandatory programme, prevalence reduction in the population might be considered a success criterion, but in a voluntary programme, the population consists only of participants that have actively decided to join the programme. Therefore, even though a targeted prevalence reduction may only include the participating herds, some of the non-participating herds may not be infected and consequently would not be a target during control efforts. Therefore, success parameters may be more difficult to establish. Participation in the Danish MAP programme peaked in the period 2009-2011, with 29% of herds enrolled, representing 36% of cows in Denmark. The between-herd prevalence in the whole country was estimated at approximately 85% (Nielsen, 2014b). Consequently, there were some herds presumed to be infected that were not enrolled. But should that be considered a failure? The programme only aimed at providing tools to reduce the within-herd prevalence for those requiring them, and as such, the goal was only to reduce prevalence in the participating herds, irrespective of how many of these there were. This goal seems to have been achieved (Nielsen and Toft, 2011). However, from an industry point of view it could be considered a failure that not all infected herds are enrolled. This is one of the questions of a voluntary programme: who should be included and what is the effect of not being able to include all herds? The answer to this question is not addressed in this book. However, a change in the status of the disease from 'potentially zoonotic' to 'proven zoonotic' would have a major effect, and would be likely to impact the entire setup and approach to control, from bottom-up to top-down, including a change of the stakeholder role played by the authorities and industry.

References

Anonymous, 2013. Bekendtgørelse om Salmonella hos kvæg mm. (BEK nr. 954 af 10/07/2013). Fødevareministeriet.

Barkema HW, Bartels CJ, van Wuijckhuise L, Hesselink JW, Holzhauer M, Weber MF, Franken P, Kock PA, Bruschke CJ, Zimmer GM, 2001. Outbreak of bovine virus diarrhea on Dutch dairy farms induced by a bovine herpesvirus 1 marker vaccine. Tijdschrift voor Diergeneeskunde 126: 158-165.

Benedictus G, Verhoeff J, Schukken YH, Hesselink JW, 2000. Dutch paratuberculosis programme history, principles and development. Veterinary Microbiology 77:399-413.

Behr MA, Kapur V, 2008. The evidence for *Mycobacterium paratuberculosis* in Crohn's disease. Current Opinions in Gastroenterology 24:17-21.

Bitsch V, Hansen K-EL, Rønsholt L, 2000. Experiences from the Danish programme for eradication of bovine virus diarrhoea (BVD) 1994–1998 with special reference to legislation and causes of infection. Veterinary Microbiology 77, 137-143.

Bitsch V, Rønsholt L, 1995. Control of bovine viral diarrhea virus infection without vaccines. Veterinary Clinics of North America. Food Animal Practice 11:627-640.

Bolin SR, McClurkin AW, Cutlip RC, Coria MF, 1985. Severe clinical disease induced in cattle persistently infected with noncytopathic bovine viral diarrhea virus by superinfection with cytopathic bovine viral diarrhea virus. American Journal of Veterinary Research, 46: 573-576.

Brownlie J, Clarke MC, Howard CJ, 1984. Experimental production of fatal mucosal disease in cattle. Veterinary Record, 114: 535-536.

Bøttner A, Belsham GJ, 2012. Virus survival in slurry: Analysis of the stability of foot-and-mouth disease, classical swine fever, bovine viral diarrhoea and swine influenza viruses. Veterinary Microbiology, 157, 41-49

Carman S, T van Dreumel, J Ridpath, M. Hazlett, D Alves, E Dubovi, R Tremblay, S Bolin, A Godkin, N Anderson. 1998. Severe acute bovine viral diarrhea in Ontario 1993-1995. Journal of Veterinary Diagnostic Investigation 10, 27-35.

Collins DM, Gabric DM, De Lisle GW, 1989. Identification of a repetitive DNA sequence specific to *Mycobacterium paratuberculosis*. FEMS Microbiology Letters 51:175-178.

Coussens P, Lamont EA, Kabara E, 2009. Chapter 11. Host-Pathogen interactions and intracellular survival of *Mycobacterium avium* subsp. *paratuberculosis*. In: Behr M and Collins DM (Eds.): Paratuberculosis. Organism, Disease and Control, p. 109-125.

Dubovi EJ, 2013. Laboratory diagnosis of bovine viral diarrhea virus. Biologicals, 41, 8-13.

Givens MD, Stringfellow DA, Dykstra CC, Riddell KP, Galik PK, Sullivan E., Robl J, Poothapillai K, Kumar A, Boykin DW, 2004. Prevention and elimination of bovine viral diarrhea virus infections in fetal fibroblast cells. Antiviral Research 64: 113-118.

Goyal SM, 2005. Diagnosis. *In*: Bovine viral diarrhea virus - diagnosis, management and control, ed. Goyal SM, Ridpath JF, pp. 197–208. Blackwell Publishing, Ames, IA.

Grimont PAD, Grimont F, Bouvet P, 2000. Taxonomy of the genus Salmonella. In: Wray, C., Wray, A. (Eds.), Salmonella in Domestic Animals. CABI Publishing, New York, pp. 1-17.

Groenendaal H, Nielen M, Hesselink JW, 2003. Development of the Dutch Johne's disease control program supported by a simulation model. Preventive Veterinary Medicine 60:69-90.

Gunn HM, 1993. Role of fomites and flies in the transmission of bovine viral diarrhoea virus. Veterinary Record 132: 584-585.

Hall GA, Jones PW, 1979. Experimental oral infections of pregnant heifers with *Salmonella* Dublin. British Veterinary Journal, 135, 75-82.

Hardman PM, Wathes CM, Wray C, 1991. Transmission of salmonellae among calves penned individually. Veterinary Record, 129, 327-329.

Hinton M, 1974. *Salmonella* Dublin Abortion in Cattle - Studies on Clinical Aspects of Condition. British Veterinary Journal, 130, 556-563.

Hirsh DC, Biberstein EL, 2004. Mycobacterium. In: Hirsh DC, MacLachlan NJ, Walker RL (Eds.). Veterinary Microbiology, 2nd Edition, Blackwell Publishing, Ames, Iowa, USA, p. 229.

Houe H, 1992. Age distribution of animals persistently infected with bovine virus diarrhoea virus (BVDV) in 22 Danish dairy herds. Canadian Journal of Veterinary Research 56: 194-198.

Houe H, 1993. Survivorship of animals persistently infected with bovine virus diarrhoea virus (BVDV). Preventive Veterinary Medicine 15: 275-283.

Houe H, 1996. Bovine virus diarrhoea virus (BVDV). Epidemiological studies of the infection among cattle in Denmark and USA. Dr.vet.med. thesis, The Royal Veterinary and Agricultural University, Copenhagen, Denmark, pp. 1-241.

Houe H, 2005. Risk Assessment. *In*: Bovine Viral Diarrhea Virus – Diagnosis, Management and Control, editors Sagar M. Goyal and Julia F. Ridpath, Blackwell Publishing, Ames, Iowa, page 35-64.

Houe H, Meyling A, 1991. Prevalence of bovine virus diarrhoea (BVD) in 19 Danish dairy herds and estimation of incidence of infection in early pregnancy. Preventive Veterinary Medicine 11: 9-16.

Houe H, Pedersen KM, Meyling A, 1993. A computerized spread sheet model for calculating total annual national losses due to bovine virus diarrhoea virus (BVDV) infection in dairy herds and sensitivity analysis of selected parameters. Proceedings of the Second Symposium on ruminant pestiviruses. 01-03 October 1992: 179-184.

House JK, Smith BP, Dilling GW, Roden LD, 1993. Enzyme-linked immunosorbent assay for serologic detection of *Salmonella* Dublin carriers on a large dairy. American Journal of Veterinary Research, 54, 1391-1399.

Jensen CO, 1891. Om den infektiøse Kalvediarrhoe og dens Aarsag. Maanedsskrift for Dyrlæger, 4: 140-162 (In Danish).

Jones PW, 1976. The effect of temperature, solids content and pH on the survival of salmonellas in cattle slurry. British Veterinary Journal 132: 284-293.

Jones PW, Smith GS, Bew J, 1977. The Effect of the microflora in cattle slurry on the survival of *Salmonella* Dublin. British Veterinary Journal, 133: 1-8.

Jordan D, Nielsen LR, Warnick LD, 2008. Modelling a national programme for the control of foodborne pathogens in livestock: the case of *Salmonella* Dublin in the Danish cattle industry. Epidemiology and Infection, 136: 1521-1536.

Katholm J, Houe H, 2006. Bovine Virus diarrhoea: Possible spread by contaminated medicine. Veterinary Record 158: 798-799.

Kjeldsen MK, Torpdahl M, Campos J, Pedersen K, Nielsen EM, 2014. Multiple-locus variable-number tandem repeat analysis of *Salmonella enterica* subsp. *enterica* serovar Dublin. Journal of Applied Microbiology, 116: 1044-1054.

Konrad H, Smith BP, Dilling GW, House JK, 1994. Production of *Salmonella* serogroup D (O9)-specific enzyme-linked immunosorbent assay antigen. American Journal of Veterinary Research 55: 1647-1651.

Kudahl AB, Nielsen SS, 2009. Effect of paratuberculosis on slaughter weight and slaughter value of dairy cows. Journal of Dairy Science 92: 4340-4346.

Kudahl AB, Nielsen SS, Østergaard S, 2008. Economy, efficacy, and feasibility of a risk-based control program against paratuberculosis. Journal of Dairy Science 91:4599-4609.

Lamont EA, Bannantine JP, Armién A, Ariyakumar DS, Sreevatsan S, 2012. Identification and characterization of a spore-like morphotype in chronically starved *Mycobacterium avium* subsp. *paratuberculosis* cultures. PLoS One. 7:e30648.

Lang-Ree JR, Vatn T, Kommisrud E, Lùken T, 1994. Transmission of bovine viral diarrhoea virus by rectal examination. Veterinary Record 135: 412-413.

Larsen AB, Merkal RS, Cutlip RC, 1975. Age of cattle as related to resistance to infection with *Mycobacterium paratuberculosis*. American Journal of Veterinary Research 36:255-257.

Lepper AW, Wilks CR, Kotiw M, Whitehead JT, Swart KS, 1989. Sequential bacteriological observations in relation to cell-mediated and humoral antibody responses of cattle infected with *Mycobacterium paratuberculosis* and maintained on normal or high iron intake. Australian Veterinary Journal 66: 50-55.

Lindberg ALE, Alenius S: 1999 Principles for eradication of bovine viral diarrhoea virus (BVDV) infections in cattle populations. Veterinary Microbiology 64: 197-222.

Lombard JE, Gardner IA, Jafarzadeh SR, Fossler CP, Harris B, Capsel RT, Wagner BA, Johnson WO, 2013. Herd-level prevalence of *Mycobacterium avium* subsp. *paratuberculosis* infection in United States dairy herds in 2007. Preventive Veterinary Medicine 108: 234-238.

Lomborg S, Agerholm JS, Jensen AL, Nielsen LR, 2007. Effects of experimental immunosuppression in cattle with persistently high antibody levels to *Salmonella* Dublin lipopolysaccharide O-antigens. BMC Veterinary Research 3: 17.

Maguire H, Cowden J, Jacob M, Rowe B, Roberts D, Bruce J, Mitchell E, 1992. An outbreak of *Salmonella* Dublin infection in England and Wales associated with a soft unpasteurized cows' milk cheese. Epidemiology and Infection 109: 389-396.

Mars MH, Bruschke CJM, van Oirschot JT, 1999. Airborne transmission of BHV1, BRSV, and BVDV among cattle is possible under experimental conditions. Veterinary Microbiology 66: 197-207.

Mateus A, Taylor DJ, Brown D, Mellor DJ, Bexiga R, Ellis K, 2008. Looking for the unusual suspects: a *Salmonella* Dublin outbreak investigation. Public Health, 122: 1321-1323.

Mitchell RM, Medley GF, Collins MT, Schukken YH, 2012. A meta-analysis of the effect of dose and age at exposure on shedding of *Mycobacterium avium* subspecies *paratuberculosis* (MAP) in experimentally infected calves and cows. Epidemiology and Infection 140: 231-246.

Momotani E, Whipple DL, Thiermann AB, Cheville NF, 1988. Role of M cells and macrophages in the entrance of into domes of ileal Peyer's patches in calves. Veterinary Pathology 25: 131-137.

NAHMS, 1997. Johne's Disease on U.S. Dairy Operations. USDA-APHIS-VS, CEAH, National Animal Health Monitoring System, Fort Collins, CO (#N245.1097).

McClurkin AW, Littledike ET, Cutlip RC, Frank GH, Coria MF, Bolin SR, 1984. Production of cattle immunotolerant to bovine viral diarrhea virus. Canadian Journal of Comparative Medicine 48: 156-161.

Moennig, V., Houe, H. and Lindberg, A., 2005. BVD control in Europe: Current status and perspectives. Animal Health Research Reviews. 6: 63-74.

Nazer AHK, Osborne AD, 1977. Experimental *Salmonella* Dublin Infection in Calves. British Veterinary Journal 133: 388-398.

Nielsen LR, 2013a. Review of pathogenesis and diagnostic methods of immediate relevance for epidemiology and control of *Salmonella* Dublin in cattle. Veterinary Microbiology 162: 1-9.

Nielsen LR, 2013b. *Salmonella* Dublin faecal excretion probabilities in cattle with different temporal antibody profiles in 14 endemically infected dairy herds. Epidemiology and Infection 141: 1937-1944.

Nielsen LR, 2013c. *Salmonella* Dublin in cattle: Epidemiology, design and evaluation of surveillance and eradication programmes. Dr.vet.med. thesis, University of Copenhagen, Denmark, pp. 1-397.

Nielsen LR, 2013d. Within-herd prevalence of *Salmonella* Dublin in endemically infected dairy herds. Epidemiology and Infection 141: 2074–2082.

Nielsen LR, Kudahl AB, Østergaard S, 2012a. Age-structured dynamic, stochastic and mechanistic simulation model of *Salmonella* Dublin infection within dairy herds. Preventive Veterinary Medicine 105: 59-74.

Nielsen LR, Schukken YH, Grohn YT, Ersbøll AK, 2004a. *Salmonella* Dublin infection in dairy cattle: Risk factors for becoming a carrier. Preventive Veterinary Medicine 65: 47-62.

Nielsen LR, Toft N, Ersbøll AK, 2004b. Evaluation of an indirect serum ELISA and a bacteriological faecal culture test for diagnosis of *Salmonella* serotype Dublin in cattle using latent class models. Journal of Applied Microbiology 96: 311-319.

Nielsen LR, Warnick LD, Greiner M, 2007. Risk factors for changing test classification in the Danish surveillance program for Salmonella in dairy herds. Journal of Dairy Science 90: 2815-2825.

Nielsen SS, 2007. Danish control programme for bovine paratuberculosis. Cattle Practice 15: 161-168.

Nielsen SS, 2008. Transitions in diagnostic tests used for detection of *Mycobacterium avium* subsp. *paratuberculosis* infections in cattle. Veterinary Microbiology 132: 274-282.

Nielsen SS, 2009a. Paratuberculosis in dairy cattle. Epidemiological studies used for design of a control programme in Denmark. Dr.vet.med. thesis. University of Copenhagen, Denmark, pp. 1-292.

Nielsen SS, 2009b. Programmes on paratuberculosis in Europe. Proceedings of the 10th International Colloquium on Paratuberculosis, p. 101-108.

Nielsen SS, 2009c. Use of diagnostics for risk-based control of paratuberculosis in dairy herds. In Practice 31: 150-154.

Nielsen SS, 2011. Dairy farmers' reasons for participation in the Danish control programme on bovine paratuberculosis. Preventive Veterinary Medicine 98: 279-283.

Nielsen SS, 2014a. Developments in diagnosis and control of bovine paratuberculosis. CAB Reviews 9, 012: 1-12.

Nielsen SS, 2014b. Developments in the Danish control program on paratuberculosis 2006-2014. Proceedings of the 4th ParaTB Forum, Parma, Italy, 21 June 2014, p. 21-26.

Nielsen SS, Jepsen ØR, Aagaard K, 2007. Control programme for paratuberculosis in Denmark. Bulletin of the International Dairy Federation 410: 23-29.

Nielsen SS, Krogh MA, Enevoldsen C, 2009. Time to the occurrence of a decline in milk production in cows with various paratuberculosis antibody profiles. Journal of Dairy Science 92: 149-155.

Nielsen SS, Toft N, 2009. A review of prevalences of paratuberculosis in farmed animals in Europe. Preventive Veterinary Medicine 88: 1-14.

Nielsen SS, Toft N, 2011. Effect of management practices on paratuberculosis prevalence in Danish dairy herds. Journal of Dairy Science 94: 1849-1857.

Nielsen TD, Kudahl AB, Østergaard S, Nielsen LR, 2013. Gross margin losses due to *Salmonella* Dublin infection in Danish dairy cattle herds estimated by simulation modelling. Preventive Veterinary Medicine, 111: 51-62.

Nielsen TD, Vesterbæk IL, Kudahl AB, Borup KJ, Nielsen LR, 2012b. Effect of management on prevention of *Salmonella* Dublin exposure of calves during a one-year control programme in 84 Danish dairy herds. Preventive Veterinary Medicine 105: 101-109.

Niskanen R, Lindberg A, Larsson B, Alenius A, 1996. Primarily BVDV-infected calves as transmitters of the infection. British Cattle Veterinary Association, Edinburgh 1996: 593-595.

OIE, Manual of Diagnostic Tests and Vaccines for Terrestrial Animals, 2004. Bovine Viral Diarrhea Chapter, 2.10.6.

Olafson P, MacCallum AD, Fox FH, 1946. An apparently new transmissible disease of cattle. Cornell Veterinarian 36: 205-213.

Olsen JE, Skov M, 1994. Genomic lineage of *Salmonella enterica* serovar Dublin. Veterinary Microbiology 40: 271-282.

Ott SL, Wells SJ, Wagner BA, 1999. Herd-level economic losses associated with Johne's disease on US dairy operations. Preventive Veterinary Medicine 40:179-192.

Payne JM, Rankin JD, 1961. The pathogenesis of experimental Johne's disease in calves. Research in Veterinary Science 2: 167–174.

Pesch KL, 1926. Meningitis durch bacterium enteritidis (Gärtner). Zentralblatt fuer Bakteriologie 98: 22-24.

Plym-Forshell L, Ekesbo I, 1996. Survival of *Salmonellas* in urine and dry faeces from cattle - An experimental study. Acta Veterinaria Scandinavica 37: 127-131.

Presi P, Struchen R, Knight-Jones T, Scholl S, Heim D, 2011. Bovine viral diarrhea (BVD) eradication in Switzerland-Experiences of the first two years. Preventive Veterinary Medicine 99: 112-121.

Raizman EA, Fetrow J, Wells SJ, Godden SM, Oakes MJ, Vazquez G, 2007. The association between *Mycobacterium avium* subsp. *paratuberculosis* fecal shedding or clinical Johne's disease and lactation performance on two Minnesota, USA dairy farms. Preventive Veterinary Medicine 78: 179-195.

Ramsey FK, Chivers WH, 1953. Mucosal Disease of Cattle. North American Veterinarian 34: 629-633.

Richardson A, 1973. The transmission of *Salmonella* Dublin to calves from adult carrier cows. Veterinary Record 92: 112-115.

Richardson A, Watson WA, 1971. A contribution to the epidemiology of *Salmonella* Dublin infection in cattle. British Veterinary Journal 127: 173-182.

Richardson E, More S, 2009. Direct and indirect effects of Johne's disease on farm and animal productivity in an Irish dairy herd. Irish Veterinary Journal 62: 526-32.

Ridpath JF, 2010. Bovine viral diarrhea virus: Global status. Veterinary Clinics of North America. Food Animal Practice 26: 105-121.

Rossmanith W, Deinhofer M, Janacek R, Trampler R, Wilhelm E, 2010. Voluntary and compulsory eradication of bovine viral diarrhoea virus in Lower Austria. Veterinary Microbiology 142: 143-149.

Rønsholt L Nylin B, Bitsch V, 1997. A BVDV antigen- and antibody blocking ELISA (DVIV) system used in a Danish voluntary eradication program. In: Proceedings of the third ESVV symposium on pestivirus infections, Lelystad, The Netherlands, 19-20 September 1996. ed. Edwards S, Paton DJ, Wensvoort G. pp. 150-153.

Saatkamp HW, Stott AW, Humphrey, RW, Gunn GJ, 2006. Socioeconomic aspects of BVDV control. *In* EU Thematic Network on Control of Bovine Viral Diarrhoea Virus (BVDV), QLRT – 2001-01573: Position Paper, pp. 99-133.

Saliki JT, Dubovi EJ, 2004, Laboratory diagnosis of bovine viral diarrhea virus infections. Veterinary Clinics of North America. Food Animal Practice 20:69–83.

Sandvik T, 2005, Selection and use of laboratory diagnostic assays in BVD control programmes. Preventive Veterinary Medicine 72: 3–16.

Sergeant ES, Nielsen SS, Toft N, 2008. Evaluation of test-strategies for estimating probability of low prevalence of paratuberculosis in Danish dairy herds. Preventive Veterinary Medicine 85: 92-106.

Segall T, Lindberg AA, 1991. Experimental oral *Salmonella* Dublin infection in calves: A bacteriological and pathological study. Journal of Veterinary Medicine B 38: 169-184.

Sojka WJ, Thomson PD, Hudson EB, 1974. Excretion of *Salmonella* Dublin by adult bovine carriers. British Veterinary Journal 130: 482-488.

Spier SJ, Smith BP, Tyler JW, Cullor JS, Dilling GW, Da Pfaff L, 1990. Use of ELISA for detection of immunoglobulins G and M that recognize *Salmonella* Dublin lipopolysaccharide for prediction of carrier status in cattle. American Journal of Veterinary Research 51: 1900-1904.

Stabel JR, 2006. Host responses to *Mycobacterium avium* subsp. *paratuberculosis*: a complex arsenal. Animal Health Research Reviews 7: 61-70.

Stevenson K, 2009. Chapter 12: Comparative differences between strains of *Mycobacterium avium* subsp. *paratuberculosis*. In: Behr M and

Collins DM (Eds.): Paratuberculosis. Organism, Disease and Control, p. 109-125.

Sweeney RW, 2011. Pathogenesis of paratuberculosis. Veterinary Clinics of North American. Food Animal Practice 27:537-546.

Sweeney RW, Whitlock RH, Rosenberger AE, 1992. *Mycobacterium paratuberculosis* cultured from milk and supramammary lymph nodes of infected asymptomatic cows. Journal of Clinical Microbiology 30: 166-171.

Steinbach G, Koch H, Meyer H, Klaus C, 1996. Influence of prior infection on the dynamics of bacterial counts in calves experimentally infected with *Salmonella* Dublin. Veterinary Microbiology 48: 199-206.

Ståhl K, Alenius S, 2012. BVDV control and eradication in Europe - an update. Japanese Journal of Veterinary Research 60: 31-39.

Tavornpanich S, Wells SJ, Fossler CP, Roussel AJ, Gardner IA, 2012. Evaluation of an alternative method of herd classification for infection with paratuberculosis in cattle herds in the United States. American Journal of Veterinary Research 73: 248-256.

Taylor AW, 1953. Experimental Johne's disease in cattle. Journal of Comparative Pathology 63: 355-367.

Taylor RJ, Burrows MR, 1971. The survival of Escherichia coli and *Salmonella* Dublin in slurry on pasture and the infectivity of *S.* Dublin for grazing calves. British Veterinary Journal: 127, 536-542.

Tarry DW, Bernal L, Edwards S, 1991. Transmission of bovine virus diarrhoea virus by blood feeding flies. Veterinary Record 128: 82-84.

Tråvén M, Alenius S, Fossum C, Larsson B, 1991. Primary bovine viral diarrhoea virus infection in calves following direct contact with a persistently viraemic calf. Journal of Veterinary Medicine B 38: 453-462.

Uttenthal Å, Stadejek T, Nylin B, 2005. Genetic diversity of bovine viral diarrhoea viruses (BVDV) in Denmark during a 10-year eradication period. Acta Pathologica Microbiologica et Immunologica Scandinavica, 113: 536-541.

Valle PS, Martin SW, Tremblay R, Bateman K, 1999. Factors associated with being a bovine-virus diarrhoea (BVD) seropositive herd in the Møre and Romsdal county of Norway. Preventive Veterinary Medicine 40:165-177.

Vaarst M, Nissen TB, Østergaard S, Klaas IC, Bennedsgaard TW, Christensen J, 2007. Danish stable schools for experiential common learning in groups of organic dairy farmers. Journal of Dairy Science 90: 2543-2554.

van Roermund HJ, Bakker D, Willemsen PT, de Jong MC, 2007. Horizontal transmission of *Mycobacterium avium* subsp. paratuberculosis in cattle in an experimental setting: calves can transmit the infection to other calves. Veterinary Microbiology 122: 270-279.

Vazquez P, Garrido JM, Juste RA, 2013. Specific antibody and interferon-gamma responses associated with immunopathological forms of bovine paratuberculosis in slaughtered Friesian cattle. PLoS One. 8: e64568.

Wallis TS, Paulin SM, Plested JS, Watson PR, Jones PW, 1995. The *Salmonella* Dublin virulence plasmid mediates systemic but not enteric phases of salmonellosis in cattle. Infection and Immunity, 63, 2755-2761.

Warnick LD, Nielsen LR, Nielsen J, Greiner M, 2006. Simulation model estimates of test accuracy and predictive values for the Danish Salmonella surveillance program in dairy herds. Preventive Veterinary Medicine 77: 284-303.

Whittington RJ, Windsor PA, 2009. In utero infection of cattle with *Mycobacterium avium* subsp. *paratuberculosis*: a critical review and meta-analysis. Veterinary Journal 179: 60-69.

Whittington RJ, Marshall DJ, Nicholls PJ, Marsh IB, Reddacliff LA, 2004. Survival and dormancy of *Mycobacterium avium* subsp. *paratuberculosis* in the environment. Applied and Environmental Microbiology 70: 2989-3004.

Whittington RJ, Marsh IB, Reddacliff LA, 2005. Survival of *Mycobacterium avium* subsp. *paratuberculosis* in dam water and sediment. Applied and Environmental Microbiology 71: 5304-5308.

Wray C, Davies RH, 2000. Salmonella infections in cattle. In: Wray, C., Wray, A. (Eds.) Salmonella in Domestic Animals. CABI Publishing, New York, New York State, pp. 169-190.

Wray C, Sojka WJ, 1981. *Salmonella* Dublin infection of calves: Use of small doses to simulate natural infection on the farm. Journal of Hygiene 87: 501-509.